Essential Skills

for Postgraduates in Dentistry

Essential Skills
for Postgraduates in Dentistry

Sabita M Ram MDS
Professor and Head, Department of Prosthetic Dentistry
Mahatma Gandhi Mission's Dental College & Hospital
Navi Mumbai, Maharashtra, India

Richard Pereira MDS FICD MBA
Professor, Department of Periodontics
Mahatma Gandhi Mission's Dental College & Hospital
Navi Mumbai, Maharashtra, India

Foreword
Prof. C. Bhasker Rao

JAYPEE The Health Sciences Publisher
New Delhi | London | Philadelphia | Panama

Jaypee Brothers Medical Publishers (P) Ltd

Headquarters

Jaypee Brothers Medical Publishers (P) Ltd
4838/24, Ansari Road, Daryaganj
New Delhi 110 002, India
Phone: +91-11-43574357
Fax: +91-11-43574314
Email: jaypee@jaypeebrothers.com

Overseas Offices

J.P. Medical Ltd
83 Victoria Street, London
SW1H 0HW (UK)
Phone: +44 20 3170 8910
Fax: +44 (0)20 3008 6180
Email: info@jpmedpub.com

Jaypee-Highlights Medical Publishers Inc
City of Knowledge, Bld. 235, 2nd Floor, Clayton
Panama City, Panama
Phone: +1 507-301-0496
Fax: +1 507-301-0499
Email: cservice@jphmedical.com

Jaypee Medical Inc
325 Chestnut Street
Suite 412, Philadelphia
PA 19106, USA
Phone: +1 267-519-9789
Email: support@jpmedus.com

Jaypee Brothers Medical Publishers (P) Ltd
17/1-B Babar Road, Block-B, Shaymali
Mohammadpur, Dhaka-1207
Bangladesh
Mobile: +08801912003485
Email: jaypeedhaka@gmail.com

Jaypee Brothers Medical Publishers (P) Ltd
Bhotahity, Kathmandu, Nepal
Phone: +977-9741283608
Email: kathmandu@jaypeebrothers.com

Website: www.jaypeebrothers.com
Website: www.jaypeedigital.com

Inquiries for bulk sales may be solicited at: jaypee@jaypeebrothers.com

Essential Skills for Postgraduates in Dentistry

First Edition: **2016**

ISBN 978-93-85999-67-3

Printed at: Samrat Offset Pvt. Ltd.

Contributors

Aditya Mitra MDS
Professor, Department of Conservative Dentistry & Endodontics
Guru Nanak Institute of Dental Sciences & Research
Panihati, Kolkata, India

Ajay Kakar MDS
Consultant Periodontist, LH Hiranandani Hospital Powai,
HON Consultant, MGM Dental College
Navi Mumbai, Mumbai, Maharastra, India
Clinical Adjunct Professor,
Stony Brook Dental School, SUNY, USA

Arun Nayak MDS
Diplomate of Indian Board of Orthodontics

Arun Sharma BDS MSC
Clinical Professor and Director, Graduate Prosthodontics
University of California, San Francisco, USA
Diplomate American Board of Prosthodontics,
Vice Chair Editorial Council for the Journal
of Prosthetic Dentistry

Munira Hirkani MBBS MD (Human Physiology)
GSMC FAIMER FELLOW & FACULTY
Associate Professor, Department of Physiology
Seth G.S Medical College & K.E.M. Hospital
Mumbai, Maharashtra, India

Richard Pereira MDS FICD MBA (Health Care)
Professor, Department of Periodontics
MGM Dental College & Hospital
Navi Mumbai, Maharashtra, India

Sabita M Ram MDS
Dean, Professor & Head, Department of Prosthodontics
MGM Dental College & Hospital
Navi Mumbai, Maharashtra, India

Seema Anjenaya MBBS MD (Community Medicine) GSMC-FAIMER FELLOW 2009
Professor & HOD, Community Medicine, Director,
MGM School of Health Management Studies, &
Member of Board of Management,
MGM Institute of Health Sciences (MGMIHS),
MGM Medical College,
Navi-Mumbai, Mumbai, Maharastra, India

Sudhindra Kulkarni MDS (Perio) DIPLOMATE (ICOI, USA)
Professor, Department of Periodontics
SDM College of Dental Sciences and Hospital
Dharwad, Karnataka, India

Sujata Kanhere MBBS DCH DNB (PEDS) MNAMS FRCPCH (LONDON) PhD
CGEIT FELLOWSHIP IN PEDIATRIC NEUROLOGY (UK)
GSMC-FAIMER FELLOW (2006) & FACULTY
Professor & Head of Unit, In charge Pediatric Neurology,
Department of Pediatrics
KJ Somaiya Medical College & Hospital,
Mumbai, Maharashtra, India

Sunita Gupta MDS MBA (HCA) FICD (USA)
COMMON WEALTH FELLOW (UK) INDO-HUNGARIAN FELLOW
Professor & Head - Oral Medicine and Radiology
Maulana Azad Institute of Dental Sciences, MAMC Campus,
New Delhi, India

Suresh Chari PhD (MED BIOCHEM) GSMC FAIMER FELLOW 2009
DIPLOMA IN PHYCOLOGIAL COUNCELLING
Soft Skills Trainer, Director Research & Medical Education
Technology and Prof Biochemistry
Director Research & MET and Professor Biochemistry
NKP Salve Institute of Medial Science & Research Center,
Nagpur, Maharastra, India

Vinayak Joshi MDS MS (Oral Biology & Pathology, USA) PhD
ASM-IUSSTF INDO-US RESEARCH PROFESSORSHIP-2011
Associate Professor, Department of Periodontology
Maratha Mandal's NGH Institute of Dental Sciences
and Research Centre, Belgaum, Karnataka, India

Foreword

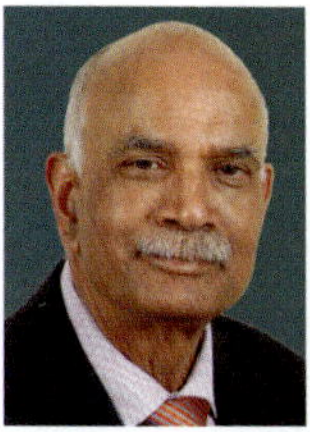

I am pleased to note the publication of this book, which should serve as a useful supplement to some of the important facets of postgraduate dental studies—reviewing articles for presentation in journal clubs and publication, preparing seminars, etc. These are aspects that are very different to what the dental graduate has previously encountered during his/her undergraduate degree programme, where the teaching programme is essentially a didactics (with notes and handouts) and chair-side clinical training. This is far from the demands of postgraduate studies, where the emphasis is more on self-reading and learning, and critical review and analysis of the evidence base. This is where "Essential Skills for Postgraduates in Dentistry" can makes a difference and I am pleased to see that the editors—whom I have known for over 15 years—have endeavored to share their experience and expertise with the postgraduate dental student. The book will be a useful addition to the new postgraduate's armamentarium and I wish Dr. Sabita M. Ram and Dr. Richard Pereira success.

Prof. C. Bhasker Rao
Former Principal and Director
SDM Dental College
Vice President, DCI

From the Author's desk...

There are over 100 odd dental institutes offering postgraduate courses in India and a clamour of students rushing into such programmes. As part of the curriculum, the first time postgraduate student is required to engage in several activities that are totally new to him/her. He is required to publish articles, prepare seminars, journal clubs, etc. without actually having a reference manual on how to do same. This handbook aims to bridge that gap by providing that information, thus creating well-informed students who are better equipped in effectively pursuing his/her course.

With this background, we decided to piece together various topics of relevance for a postgraduate student in his programme and then approached experts in their respective fields to contribute. We were fortunate to be blessed by enthusiastic contributors/teachers of repute to be part of this academic exercise and we thank them for their support..

We also intend this book to be used by medical postgraduates as most of the topics are broad-based and can be adapted to their postgraduate programme as well. We do sincerely hope that our students find this manual informative, concise and helpful.

We also believe that a teacher should be a guide by the side rather than a sage on the stage for every student and that every student should have a mind that is perpetually yearning to learn and hone one's skills. This book is dedicated to all such students !

Sabita M Ram
Richard Pereira

Preface

Maximizing the Postgraduate Program

The Proactive Postgraduate Student

INTRODUCTION

As a postgraduate (PG), student, one enters their PG program with a lot of trepidation not knowing what to really expect. A student comes in with a mindset of a graduate student unsure of what lies ahead. A PG program is a lot more demanding, requires a lot more commitment, dedication and hard work to produce the results one desires. It requires, besides the cognitive skills, an attitudinal shift to be able to grapple with the challenges that lie ahead. That shift in mindset is the first and foremost need to begin with.

SET YOUR GOALS

Goal setting is a very important exercise in life and especially in the PG program ahead; it helps give your mind a certain direction. Without goals it would be like placing your ladder against a tree, climbing to the top and then realizing you're against the wrong tree. So first decide which tree you want to climb.

At different junctures the program ahead will offer you several options and opportunities, so only a clear mindset at every decision will help you decide ahead. Your goals should be SMART; Specific Measurable, Attainable, Result oriented and Time bound. Being specific and laser focused helps the mind achieve clarity; the goal ahead should be practical, measurable and something that can be attained in a fixed time frame. Once the goal is decided, never change the goal post but only the route to the goal if you have to! Success in your course is based on 3 keys, the information you harness, the people you spend time with and the action you take. So taking action on the goals you set is fundamental to success.

HONE PERIPHERAL SKILL SETS

Practice management is never taught in dental college but it is wise to master your skills of patient communication, record keeping and treatment analysis with patients as that form the essence of your practice in the future.

TIME SCHEDULING

Get into a habit of mapping out your activities into ones that productive ones and non-productive ones. You will be surprised how much time is spent on useless ones. It's like a leaky bucket where time is just simply lost and your not even aware of it. Noting down your schedules allows one to fine tune your time which can be very precious especially in the final year of the program.

ALTITUDE IS THROUGH RIGHT "ATTITUDE"

Opportunities are either NO WHERE or NOW HERE, depending on how you see it. Whatever you decide to take up strive to be the best in it. Remember to get on top; you have to get off your bottom first. And this means hard work and dedication and commitment to the goal set. At this point I would love to stress on "Attitude"; Altitude is through Attitude alone and having the right attitude is fundamental. Inculcating in one's self-discipline of time management, work ethics and integrity goes a long way in churning out the same approach in the future. Very often we see this same attitude go downhill during the first year of the PG program as a carefree feeling sets in as there seems to be "a lot of time' to do things. Nipping this in the bud will create in you a responsible professional with the same culture in the future!

STAY CONNECTED AND DIVERSIFY YOUR NETWORKS

Life is not all about being confined to your department and life within. When opportunities arise through conferences to move out of the 'well' go out there in to the world and connect with others. Don't be a cave dweller or stick like wall paper to your department and fellow colleagues, network with others from other institutes and you will learn a lot from them and about their professions as well. Meet with dealers, faculty from outside and broaden your contact sphere.

BEING PROACTIVE

Being proactive means being able to anticipate what the future will be, and to react accordingly before it actually happens.
Students who are proactive:

- Look at themselves and ask questions.
- Examine critically how they might perform those tasks more efficiently.
- Try to prevent problems from ever arising.
- Develop a mindset that looks to solve problems instead of dwelling on them.
- Know how to prioritize

You can be "proactive or "reactive" in your workplace, home or college.

A reactive person will say, "I get chest pains and numbness in my arm. May be I will go to the doctor." A proactive person will say, "Even though I have no symptoms, I want to live a long, healthy life so I will follow life-long habits of healthy eating and regular exercise." Yet there are times, when it is appropriate to be reactive. Sometimes one needs to be flexible to the changing needs of the environment.

The following are key behaviors that have been identified in being 'proactive'. These are the 5 P's:

1. Predict
2. Prevent
3. Plan
4. Participate
5. Perform

Predict

Learn to anticipate problems and events. Understand how things work; look for patterns; recognize the regular routines, daily practices and natural cycles that exist in your course. Use your creativity when anticipating future outcomes. Do not simply expect the past to always be a predictor for the future; use your logic. Come up with alternate scenarios for how events could happen.

Prevent

Try to look for likely and potential obstacles and problems that may occur in the future and find ways to overcome them before they become insurmountable. When you have challenges, take control and confront them head-on before they become major issues.

Plan

Proactive people always plan for the future. Look at the future and anticipate the issues and obstacles that are likely to emerge. Take steps that will bring you to a decision and will ensure success. Note all that needs to be done to achieve what you have set goals for in the future.

Participate

Be an active participant rather than an idle observer. Interact with people and be involved with whatever you are doing. Proactive people always take initiative and are part of the solution. Exert your influence and make a contribution.

Perform

Proactive people always take timely and effective action. Do not procrastinate. Whatever needs to be done should be done 'now'. Take ownership of your actions and be accountable to yourself. Proactive people take thoughtful steps to achieve what they want. They are not impulsive and do not react to the environment.

Take Responsibility of your life. Use Proactive Language – "I can," "I will," "I prefer," etc.

Ten Tips to be Proactive

1. Be organized
2. Be positive
3. Work at getting results
4. Overcome fears
5. Pay attention
6. Have confidence
7. Talk and communicate
8. Interact
9. Celebrate victory and success
10. Be enthusiastic.

AIM FOR SUCCESS

- ☐ Success is getting the best out of you, gaining respect, controlling stress and leading a happy, calm and fulfilling life.

- ☐ We try to solve our problems by looking for external solutions only to get frustrated when the problems persist. But the real solution lies within us.
- ☐ Success happens from the "inside-out".
- ☐ For having a fulfilling, joyful and successful life it is essential to:

BE: Be yourself. Know what is most important to you. Know what makes you unique.

DO: Do things that you are good at. Use your expertise in ways that help others.

HAVE: Have a life centered on what' is most important to you.

Instead of "Having" as your primary goal and then "Doing" and "Being" it is always satisfying and fruitful when you "BE", "DO" and "HAVE".

THINK LIKE A WINNER

Every student wants to be a winner and come out with flying colors in their program. Deep down, each of them wants to be successful—to "win" at life in general. Many believe they are worthy of it and deserve to win. However, majority of them are confused and disappointed that true success has not come their way.

There is a process to becoming successful. Just as there is a process to become a successful doctor, engineer or lawyer; several years of serious study and hard work- there is a process to become successful in life.

To become a winner one needs to "Think like a Winner". If you harbor thoughts of failure then all your actions will result in failure. However, if you have thoughts that are positive and about "success" you will be a winner. You need to have empowering beliefs that the world's super achievers have that makes them so successful.

There are no magic powers that make a person successful. Average people are average only to the extent they have average "thoughts" dominating their subconscious mind. Likewise successful and exceptional people are successful only to the extent they have successful and exceptional "thoughts" dominating their subconscious mind.

Whenever a negative thought enters your mind, immediately cancel it out with a positive thought.

Always imagine yourself as succeeding with God's help and believe in yourself. Keep on learning, growing and improving yourself. And finally remember that only determination, dedication, discipline and the right attitude will lead you to success in your PG program.

Richard Pereira

Contents

1

Postgraduate Seminars

Honing Your Teaching Skills

Munira Hirkani

Outline of Topics Covered

- Introduction
- What is a seminar?
- What is the role of the student?
- What is the role of a teacher?
- What is the purpose of student–led seminar?
- How do I prepare for the seminar?

INTRODUCTION

The most effective way to learn is to teach someone else.

This chapter will enable the reader to adopt practices to nurture their teaching and presentation skills in a seminar.

WHAT IS A SEMINAR?

The term Seminar is used in varied context. Student-led seminar means a meeting of a small group of people led by a student, which consists of a presentation followed by a discussion focussed on predefined topic.

WHAT IS THE ROLE OF THE STUDENT?

- As a seminar leader—to prepare and present the topic to the group. The presentation kicks off the discussion.
- As a group member—to contribute information, opinions and ask questions.

WHAT IS THE ROLE OF A TEACHER?

The teacher's role is that of a facilitator to encourage contributions from the small group by asking questions that stimulate further discussion. They may summarize the discussion and define areas of further reading.

WHAT IS THE PURPOSE OF A STUDENT-LED SEMINAR?

The word Seminar is derived from the Latin word *seminarium*, referring to a nursery, where seeds are sown to produce plants for transplanting. The seminar is targeted at providing a fertile ground for the student to learn and clarify concepts through discussion.

HOW DO I PREPARE FOR THE SEMINAR?

Some Practical Tips: Remember to **PEE** (**P**repare, **E**xecute and **E**valuate).

Prepare

- Research the topic allotted
  - Be thorough.
  - Identify the resources seeking guidance from your teachers/mentors.
- Reference all the important information; this will save time when you need to look up some information later.
- Define the objectives of your presentation.
- Filter all the relevant information to be used in your presentation.

Presenting a seminar provides the student an opportunity to:	
✓ attain a higher level of understanding ✓ internalise the material researched ✓ share ideas with other experts in the field	**Subject-related skills**
✓ hone their presentation and teaching skills ✓ enhance their communication skills ✓ collaborate ✓ deal with conflicting opinions ✓ formulate an argument ✓ build confidence ✓ learn time management ✓ develop responsibility for their own learning	**Transferable skills**

- ☐ Structure: organize and arrange the content so as to make it logical and meaningful.
- ☐ Select the audiovisual aid (AV aid) which would be apt for delivering your presentation.
  - Check for the availability of the AV aid. Use technology to aid your teaching and presentation not as a crutch without which you stumble.
- ☐ Refine your presentation to make it interesting
  - Use a bait: plan the start of your presentation interestingly to set induction, i.e. getting the audience ready and thinking about the session. This will hook the attention of the audience and reel them in. This could be as simple as beginning the presentation with a relevant case discussion to stress the importance of the topic.
  - Timing: Remember the attention span of the audience is not more than 15–20 minutes. So enhance your presentation with some interesting visuals, videos or some thought-provoking questions between the segments. Stick to the allotted time.

- Use visuals/videos to
  - illustrate key points.
  - emphasize verbal message.
  - focus audience attention.
  - stimulate audience interest.

❑ For preparing PowerPoint slides or overhead projector transparencies, follow these guidelines:

- Use a clear, easily readable font.
  - Preferably San serif font like **Arial Rounded MT Bold**, AvantGarde Md BT, Helvetica for PowerPoint slides.
  - Use typed script. A running hand is difficult to read.
- Use a type size of 54 for the title and 20 points or greater for the text.
- Text color
  - Use a light text on a dark background for slides for PowerPoint slides.
  - Use dark colors for text with OHP transparencies.
- No lengthy sentences
  - Bullet the key words and phrases.
  - Stick to one idea per slide or transparency.
  - Be a miser—limit the use of words.
  - **Follow the Rule of 7:** not more than seven lines on a slide and not more than seven words in a line.
- Avoid patterned backgrounds as they distract the attention from the main content.
- Do not make your slides and transparencies into a rainbow of colors. Make use of a maximum of three colors.
- Use highlights only for emphasising a particular point.
- Spare the PowerPoint slides from undue animation and sound effects.

- ☐ Include the recent advances and clinical application of a particular topic, especially when the seminar is meant for postgraduate students.
- ☐ Rehearsing the presentation will
  - familiarize you with the teaching materials created
  - aid you in verbalizing the explanations to be put forth.
  - assist you in coordinating the verbal delivery of the content with your teaching materials.
  - give you an idea of the timing to be maintained for the various sections.
- ☐ Inform the audience regarding the venue and time in advance.

Execute

Before the Seminar

- ☐ If using a PowerPoint carry a copy of the presentation with all media included on a pen-drive.
- ☐ Check out the venue of the seminar and the AV aids in advance to prevent last moment hassles.

During the Seminar

- ☐ Be calm and present confidently.
- ☐ Define the objectives of the seminar at the start and give a brief overview of your plan for it.
- ☐ Verbal communication.
  - Find your voice
  - Project your voice
  - Speak clearly
  - Pace your talk—do not speak too fast just to complete the presentation. Short pauses in between help you to gather your thoughts and also regain audience attention.

- Emphasize an important point by varying your speech rate, pitch or tone.

- ☐ Non-verbal communication: body language is a key element in the art of delivering a good oral presentation. Most of the problems associated with body language can be rectified if you carefully study yourself in a mirror.
  - Do not hide behind the podium.
  - Talk to the audience: maintain eye contact with most of the audience. Avoid addressing only those you are comfortable with.
  - Vary your facial expressions: this will add meaning and energy to what you want to convey.
  - Stance speaks: maintain a balanced stance with weight evenly distributed but lean slightly forward to show that you are engaged with the audience. Your stance conveys your ease and enthusiasm. Do not fold your arms during the presentation.
  - Use gestures to make a point, but do not go overboard with their use.
  - When not gesturing, place your hands by your side. This projects ease. Moving constantly or making a movement repetitively may annoy and distract the audience.
- ☐ Teaching with technology: use AV aids effectively. While using them confirm their visibility and audibility to the audience. Do not stand so that the screen is obscured
- ☐ Answer questions politely. Do not become defensive. Be open to different ideas and viewpoints. Formulate arguments coherently and support replies with references wherever possible.
- ☐ Do summarize the points discussed at the end.
- ☐ Appropriately acknowledge all those who have contributed to the seminar.
- ☐ Share the references used.

- Finish well within the allotted time, so as to provide time for discussion which will provide value addition to your seminar.
- Seek feedback on content, presentation skills and teaching skills; accept feedback positively to change for the better.

Evaluate

Self reflection: reflect on your overall presentation and delivery skills. Ask a colleague to video record the seminar. This will also help you evaluate your own performance critically, so as to hone your teaching skills.
Feedback from teachers and peers: seek feedback verbally or more formally using a feedback evaluation form. A sample form is printed below.

"Teaching and presenting is a skill which can only improve with practice and incorporating the feedback to improve it."

SUGGESTED READING

1. Brown G. & Manogue M. (2001) AMEE Medical Education Guide No.22: Refreshing lecturing: a guide for lecturers. *Medical Teacher*, 23: 231-244.
2. Farrow R. ABC of learning and teaching in medicine-*Creating teaching materials.* BMJ. 2003 April 26; 326: 921-923.
3. Hirkani M & Dandekar S., Large Group Teaching: Lecture as a teaching tool. In. Bhuiyan PS, Rege NN, Supe AN (Eds) *The Art of Teaching Medical Students*, 3 rd edition, 2015; 135-145 Elsevier Publishers.

SEMINAR EVALUATION FORM

Student: Date:
Topic: Evaluator:

Rating: 1=never 2=rarely 3=sometimes 4=most of the times 5=always

- Please rate the seminar for the areas mentioned below
- Comment on:
  1. What was done well 2. What could be done better

1. Content	**1**	**2**	**3**	**4**	**5**
Concepts and information presented were relevant to the topic. Content matched audience's needs.					
Comments:					
2. Critical thinking skills	**1**	**2**	**3**	**4**	**5**
Cited current literature. Made connections between different ideas. Constructed and justified answers. Solved problems in a systematic manner.					
Comments:					
3. Communication skills	**1**	**2**	**3**	**4**	**5**
Organized content logically. Explained information clearly. Maintained eye contact, speech was clear and well-spaced, used correct language.					
Comments:					
4. Ability to respond to queries	**1**	**2**	**3**	**4**	**5**
Answered accurately with the expected level of competence. Answered non- defensively. Supported answers with relevant references.					
Comments:					
5. Use of Audiovisual aid	**1**	**2**	**3**	**4**	**5**
Used appropriate AV aid. Used them effectively					
Comments:					
6. Interaction with the audience	**1**	**2**	**3**	**4**	**5**
Asked questions, allowed questions from the audience, made clarifications					
Comments:					

Modified from *https://www.utexas.edu/pharmacy/general/experiential/practitioner/formal.pdf (last accessed on 10 September 2015).*

2

Journal Clubs

The Art of Analysis

Arun Sharma

Outline of Topics Covered

- Why have Journal Clubs?
- How to evaluate the scientific literature?
- How do you start to read an article?
- Quality of the Journal

WHY HAVE JOURNAL CLUBS?

Critically analyzing scientific articles is not something most people are taught during their professional training. The first exposure to critically reading and analyzing an article starts during a masters or residency program. Just because an article has been published, it does not mean that what is presented is accurate and validated. Critically analyzing the scientific literature is an art, because it takes experience and time to develop this skill. Journal clubs play a very important role in developing this skill. The mentor leading the discussion has the advantage of having read some of the articles more than once.

A journal club session needs to be devoted to one topic (e.g. squamous cell carcinoma of the maxillary sinus). Before you start discussing the individual article you should outline the questions you would like to have answered by the end of the discussion.

- What do I want to know about this topic?—Diagnosis, incidence, risk factors, clinical management, reconstruction, prognosis.
- As you review each article, make sure you are able to answer the questions you wanted answered.
- At the end of the session, summarize the conclusions of all the articles and make sure you know which article answered the question you had set out to answer.

HOW TO EVALUATE THE SCIENTIFIC LITERATURE?

Objective

- To be able to critically read and evaluate information presented in the literature as it pertains to practice.
- Knowledge of classical and current literature in preparation for a master's degree or speciality board examination.

There are two sources of inaccurate information involved in deciphering scientific articles:

- Information presented may be erroneous or inaccurate.
- Information in the article may be misinterpreted by the reader.

The journal club should assist you in analyzing both the writer's ability to convey information, and your ability to critically read and evaluate the information presented.

Classification of Articles

All articles can be classified into two categories:

1. Reports: In general, reports convey information that cannot be critically analyzed.

   a. Textbooks: broad generalizations, overviews of subject.
   b. Case reports: unusual clinical cases.
   c. Abstracts: summary.
   d. Review of literature articles: chronological summary of articles.
   e. Conference proceedings .
   f. Technique or procedure reports.
2. Experiments: They can and should be critically analyzed.
   a. Animal
   b. *In vitro*
   c. Clinical surveys

Articles from this category should represent clear thinking and logical progression of thought, leading to conclusive statements based on rational inference about the topic under question. In reading these articles identify the following:

- ☐ The problem: is it clearly stated?
- ☐ The objectives: clearly defined, hypotheses stated?
- ☐ Method: sample, design, data, statistics.
- ☐ Results
- ☐ Discussion
- ☐ Conclusions: Are conclusions warranted by the findings? Are conclusions relevant to the situation you wish to apply them to?

HOW DO YOU START TO READ AN ARTICLE?

Most scientific articles today are published with an abstract. Ignore the abstract. If you start by reading the abstract you run the risk of being biased or manipulated by what the author thinks is significant. Read the article with an open mind not any preconceived idea. Start by identifying if the article is a report or experiment. For articles in the "experiment" category make sure they follow the "Six Rules". While you are reading underline or highlight what you think is significant and also identify erroneous conclusions. Then go back and write a short summary: for "experiments" use the six categories. Do this on digital or analog 3x5 cards. During the journal club, use the reverse side of the card to make notes of the discussion. This will help when you are reviewing the papers for an examination as you will not have the time to read all the articles again. I do not like reading articles that have been underlined or highlighted by someone else—this sets up an unconscious bias and does not allow you to form your own conclusions.

QUALITY OF THE JOURNAL

It is very important to understand the review process that a journal uses before an article is accepted for publication. Is the journal an "open access" (the author pays to have his/her article published) journal. For a referred journal, the editor usually does a quick review to see if the article will be of interest to the readership and if the article has been written in the format required for publication. The editor will then send the article anonymously to at least two reviewers who are considered to be experts in the field. If statistics are involved, the article will also be reviewed by a statistician to ensure that the appropriate statistical tests were used and if the sample size, data and results are appropriate. Non referred journals do not follow this rigorous process for publication.

The "impact factor" of a journal is also a measure that is used to assess the quality of the journal. The higher the impact factor the higher the quality. The journal "Nature" has one of the highest impact factors. In many academic institutions, this measure is used in promotions for their faculty. The impact factor of a journal is a measure reflecting the average number of citations to recent articles published in that journal. It is frequently used as a proxy for the relative importance of a journal within its field, with journals with higher impact factors deemed to be more important than those with lower ones.

Recently Google Scholar has also been used to evaluate the quality of a publication. Google Scholar aims to rank articles the way researchers do, weighing the full text of each article, where it was published, who it was written by, as well as how often and how recently it has been cited in other scholarly literature.

3

Communication Skills

Bridging the Gap with Your Patients

Suresh Chari

Outline of Topics Covered

- Introduction
- Need for efective comnuication
- What is effective communication?
- The bad communicator
- The mindsets
- It is a matter of choice

INTRODUCTION

As per Charles Fletcher "aim of a physician should be to cure sometimes, relieve often and comfort always."

The challenge is to build a "trustworthy" relationship with the patient while we are curing, relieving or comforting. In fact I would not hesitate to mention that a doctor of health sciences is a "human first" and then a healer, since well-said words more often than not complete the healing process.

The challenge is even more stiff for the second line in a hospital, i.e. the residents and the third line, i.e. paramedics and other ancillary staff, since they are the "face" of the hospital and the focal point in any healthcare system.

So let us just talk about sensible, sensitive and assertive communication of postgraduates in a healthcare set up with their stakeholders: patients, relatives, peer and colleagues. The following pages are not any kind of preaching or a do's and don'ts list of effective communication. Read on and find for yourself where you stand in dealing with doctor-patient relationship. Most of the pointers are self-explanatory. This chapter is important at this point of time, since I personally believe that we all need to alter our strategies of communication to rebuild slowly yet steadily the declining patient trust.

NEED FOR EFECTIVE COMMUNICATION

The Preamble. The story: Read this real story that inspired me to work on communication workshops for doctors and if you see yourself as a doctor somewhere, then its time to rethink on your strategies of communication.

My brother's wife missed a step on the stairs, slipped and fell. Her yell told us that her back hurt and it was 8 pm of Saturday night. My father, who knew many doctors in the city came to our rescue and as any other concerned father told my brother, "let's put her on the backseat of our car and drive down to Dr A. He is the best and I know him well. He is in our club and without contacts you know how things will be at the hospital. Come quickly and make her lie down in the car."

My brother looked concerned but he did what dad said and took his place next to his wife. While in the car, my brother found courage and said "No, not him! Not Dr A. He may be the best in the field and he may be in your club and known to you. He is too damn arrogant. Has someone told him that a senior and popular doctor should not smile! No, never him. There are other options today. Dad, in your time there was only one or two at the 'top' in this speciality. Today there are many at the 'top' and I am paying for treatment and not to get humiliated. What's the use of the knowledge and skill if there is no courtesy to speak? After all they have become big and popular because of patients, then why should we be at the receiving end?"

My father silently took the turn that took them to Dr B.

Story is self-explanatory.

WHAT IS EFFECTIVE COMMUNICATION?

Communication becomes effective when you get your desired response from the receiver. Hence, I am a strong advocate of the fact that receiver is more important than a sender, since ultimately it is the receiver who will decide if your communication has been effective or ineffective because he is the one who is giving the desired response.

So let us look from the receivers' (patients') perspective. What does he expect? What type of communication does your patient prefer?

The Ten patient's Expectation Pointers

Let us take this ten-point self-check. Be honest when you say "yes" or "no" to the following.

1. I introduce myself, when I meet my patient for the first time.
2. During subsequent meeting my patient recognizes me by my name.
3. I approach my patient warmly, generally with a smile.
4. My patients find me easy to talk to.
5. I keep my language and questions with my patients simple.
6. During conversation, I care for my patients feelings.
7. I am aware of my gesture, sitting position, eye contact, face expression and phrases I use during my conversation with my patients.

8. I listen carefully to my patients and look for non- verbal cues.
9. I generally repeat what my patient says.
10. When I am with my patient, I am totally with him/her.

If you say "yes" for all the above then your communication with your patient is effective. And its time to correct any "no" as an answer. All ten are self-explanatory and you will realize each one is a communication skill.

Characteristics of Effective Communication

- Pointers 1 and 2 : A good appropriate opening.
- Pointers 3 and 4: Creating a nonthreatening environment.
- Pointer 5: Using receiver-friendly simple language.
- Pointer 6: Understanding emotions (empathizing).
- Pointer 7: Assertive communication skills.
- Pointer 8, 9 and 10: Active listening skills.

Use these every time you encounter a patient. "Every time" may sound difficult, since there are some difficult patients and relatives in certain situations. But the only pointer that has to be used more carefully in such encounters is number 7, i.e. being assertive, which means being firm yet polite. You have an option of becoming aggressive which is tempting as it gives quick results, but we would never recommend that style. You may get fast results being aggressive with difficult patients and relatives, but you will definitely loose on relationships.

Another pointer that may seem difficult is number 6, i.e. understanding emotions (empathy). Let me make it simple. Empathy is the skill of feeling what the patient feels without the patient telling you! Empathy is "feeling with" the patient while sympathy is "feeling for" the patient. Empathy is a cerebral response while sympathy is a visceral response. Once you master this skill as an art, you will start communicating with ease because we know exactly how the patient would feel when you speak or when you don't speak. You will know which language to speak and your communication will be both sensitive and sensible. You will also be calmer and have less stress.

Active listening is keeping distractions to the minimum while listening. It also means paying attention even if you disagree and being nonjudgmental. A good listener demonstrates that he is actively listening by giving nonverbal signals, which also tells the receiver that the sender is open to new thoughts and ideas. It is a good idea to give space and repeat (paraphrase) what the receiver says while in conversation. I strongly recommend training yourself to be a good listener since active listening is the strongest element to make your communication effective. Think that "only a good receiver can be a good sender."

If you train yourself to master active listening' you are actually good at empathy and hence, will in natural course of time reject aggression and adapt to assertive communication. The result of all these is that you are able to create a nonthreatening environment that is conducive for effective communication.

The Ten Benefits of Effective Communication

Why are the above ten pointers important?

1. Help in good, complete and accurate diagnosis.
2. Increases patient satisfaction.
3. Decrease patient anxiety.
4. Minimize conflicts.
5. Helps understand emotions of the patients so that you could respond accordingly.
6. Ensures that advice is followed correctly.
7. Improve "trust" in doctor-patient relationship.
8. Makes the patient feel confident to come back to you.
9. Increase the feel-good factor.

10. Heal the patient faster.

THE BAD COMMUNICATOR

You will know you are not doing well in communication with your patient if your patient's inner voice is saying one or all of these:

- ☐ Please talk to me.
- ☐ Please allow me also to talk.
- ☐ Please listen to me.
- ☐ Please tell me what you are going to do.
- ☐ Please tell me what to do.
- ☐ Please tell me how to do it.
- ☐ Please do not shout at me.
- ☐ Please tell me you understand.
- ☐ Please be patient with me.
- ☐ Please treat me as a human.

If your patient is saying any one of them, then you are a bad communicator.

Quite understandably no patient would like any doctor who:

- ☐ Does not talk properly.
- ☐ Does not listen.
- ☐ Does not give information.
- ☐ Does not show concern or respect.
- ☐ Does not treat patients as human.

THE MINDSETS

If all this is so simple to understand then why do some doctors behave the way they behave?

Here are a few mindsets:

- ☐ That's how we should be with them (patients), or else they will sit on our heads.
- ☐ Never been taught how to talk during my undergraduate

or postgraduate curriculum. This skill training was missing from my syllabus.

- ☐ My senior or teacher was always like that and they have been successful.
- ☐ Why should I change? I am what I am.
- ☐ We are doctors. We should be strict, serious, aggressive and should not become personal with the patients.

So its all in the mind. And it's time we change our mindsets.

IT IS A MATTER OF CHOICE

You can take the horse to the water but cannot make it drink.

Read the ten patient expectation pointers and the ten benefits of effective communication again slowly and surely you will realize the importance of being effective in communication is simple. It's a skill that can be learnt. But whether to learn or not is an attitude. It's your personal choice and desire to do so and to be so. If you think it's important, you will implement the ten-patient expectation pointers.

CONCLUSION

You are human first. They are human first. So we all need to be treated as humans first. So communicate effectively and that humaneness will enhance your relationship with your patient.

4

Clinical Photography

Your Eye to the Clinical World

Arun Nayak

Outline of Topics Covered

- Introduction
- Selecting a camera and accessories
- Basics of photographic exposure
- Clinical photography
- Tabletop photography
- Common errors in dental photography

INTRODUCTION

Photography as a tool is now an essential extension of any postgraduate (PG) armamentarium. As a future clinician, it is mandatory for a PG student to learn using a camera and to master clinical photography skills for the following reasons:

- Documentation of records for medico-legal reasons.
- To compare pretreatment and post treatment results.
- To document findings that may be unique and to share those findings with peers.
- For obtaining data to make presentations and teaching students.
- To use data in clinical practice for patient information and motivation.
- What we learn today is because of the clinical photographs we see in textbooks. These were available courtesy the

efforts of those authors. The profession will be furthered and our next generation will learn if you as torchbearers of your subject make that same effort.

SELECTING A CAMERA FOR CLINICAL PHOTOGRAPHY

Important Factors to Consider while Buying a Camera

- Decide your budget.
  - If you need a professional DSLR camera with a macro lens and ring flash, it will cost ₹ 60,000 or more today. Such a camera is an excellent investment for the long-term for consistent and extremely professional, textbook-quality pictures. They offer interchangeability of lenses and full manual controls.
  - If you are a camera novice or you have a gadget phobia, even an automatic point and shoot (compact zoom) camera is good enough for documentation.
  - Prosumer cameras occupy the space in terms of cost and quality between DSLRs and compact zoom cameras. They offer manual controls but no interchangeability of lenses.
  - Lenses commonly accompanying DSLR camera kits are zoom lenses [e.g. 18–55mm (~3x), 18–105 mm (~6x)]. All point and shoot cameras have zoom lenses built into them (e.g. 4x , 6x, 20x zoom). Do keep in mind that an 18–105 mm lens at 105 mm focal length is NOT THE SAME as an 105 mm macro lens. Macro lenses of Tamron (90 mm) and Sigma (105 mm) cost a third of their Nikkor (105 mm) and Canon (100 mm) counterparts.
  - Dual flashes like Nikon R1 and R2 are also excellent macro flashes.
- Be the boss when your browse

With the vast range of features and models and brands available, it becomes difficult to choose a camera on the floor of the store. Use websites like *www.dpreview.com* to help you narrow your choice of cameras to 1-2 models and then go ahead buy it.

- Look at flash position for point and shoot cameras:
  - Prefer flash position at left or right of the lens or at 11 o' clock or 1 o' clock position relative to the lens **(Fig. 4.1)**.
  - Avoid flash at 12 o' clock position **(Fig. 4.2)**.

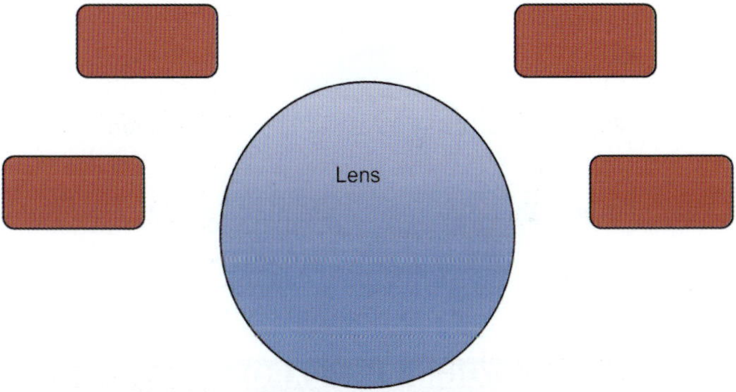

Fig. 4.1: Acceptable position of camera flashes

- Moderate zoom of upto 4x is good enough for clinical photography.
- Prefer a camera that offers aperture and shutter speed controls, RAW image capability.
- Do not worry about megapixels
  - A 4 in x 6 in print requires approximately 2 MP resolution images.
  - Any camera that offers unto 6 MP is good enough for clinical documentation.

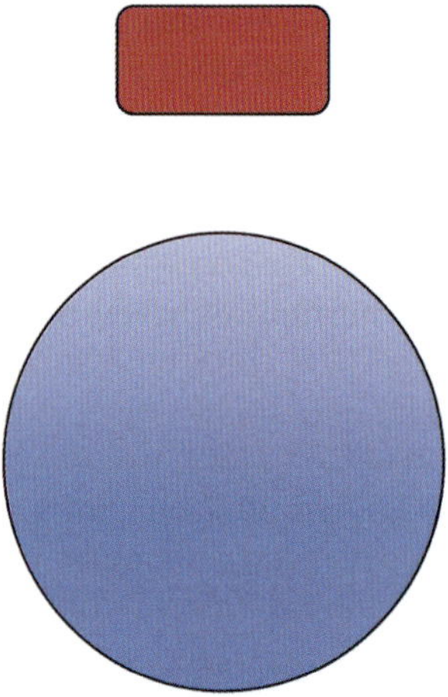

Fig. 4.2: Avoid camera flash at 12'o clock position

- ☐ Remember that to take the high quality, textbook pictures, the right equipment is mandatory, but using your photography skills, you can make a fair clinical documentation with just about any camera.

BASICS OF PHOTOGRAPHIC EXPOSURE

- ☐ A clinical photograph should have the following properties.
    - Subject should be captured "optimally", with nothing excess that may divert attention from the subject yet no part of the subject should be left-out.
    - All parts of the subject should be in "sharp" focus with no blurring.
    - All parts of the subject should be in "good light". Shadows should not obliterate any part of the subject.
    - Composition rule-of-third that may apply to creative photography, does not apply to clinical photography. "Subject should be centred" in the photograph.

- Subject should be "well-isolated".
- Alignment of the subject should be pleasing and easily interpretable.

To achieve the above objectives, you should learn

- ☐ How to use flash with respect to its intensity and position.
- ☐ Using camera controls to achieve high-resolution pictures with optimal sharpness, brightness and no shadows.

Fortunately, clinical photography involves a subject that is generally within the photographer's field of control; unlike say, wildlife photography where the subject may appear and disappear in a fraction of a second.

Light conditions in clinical photography too are under the photographer's control unlike say, outdoors photography where a sudden cloud cover can dramatically reduce light of a sunny day.

You can thereby employ these advantages of time and light to compose a good clinical photograph having all the above-mentioned properties.

USING FLASH FOR CLINICAL PHOTOGRAPHY

Flash is an integral part of clinical photography. Every kind of light is associated with a temperature. The warmer the light, the lower the temperature **(Fig. 4.3)**.

What is highly relevant to us is that Midday sun or daylight and camera flashes have the same temperature. This means that using camera flash is equivalent to using daylight akin to photographing your subject the way you see it in daylight in its most natural colors.

Flash also tends to override any other ambient light that may be present in your operatory. Therefore, in terms of quality of light, flash of the camera serves the best.

In terms of quantity, one should keep in mind that distance of the flash from the subject can alter the saturation of the colors of your subject.

Candle flame	1,500
Incandescent	3,000
Sunrise, sunset	3,500
Midday sun, flash	5,500
Bright sun, clear sky	6,000
Cloudy sky, shade	7,000
Blue sky	9,000

Fig. 4.3: Temperatures associated with light

In the following example, one can see how a small flash-subject distance and therefore high intensity of flash tends to reduce the saturation of the subject colors **(Fig. 4.4)**.

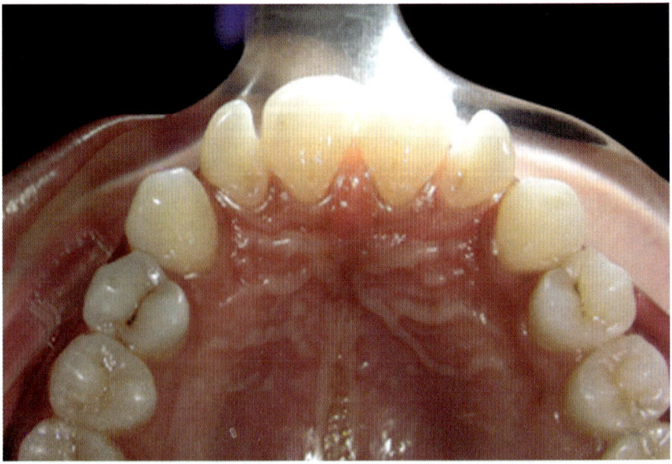

Fig. 4.4: Flash too close can destroy color and other details

To correct this problem, move away from the subject, so that light falls evenly on the subject **(Fig. 4.5)** and then crop into the subject **(Fig. 4.6)**.

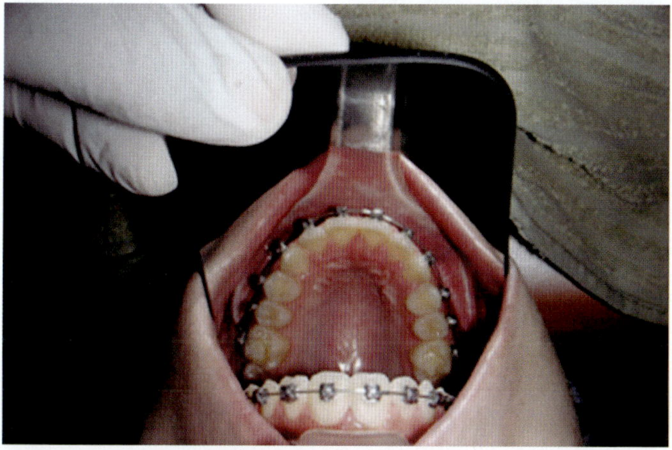

Fig. 4.5: Increasing subject-camera distance gives uniform illumination

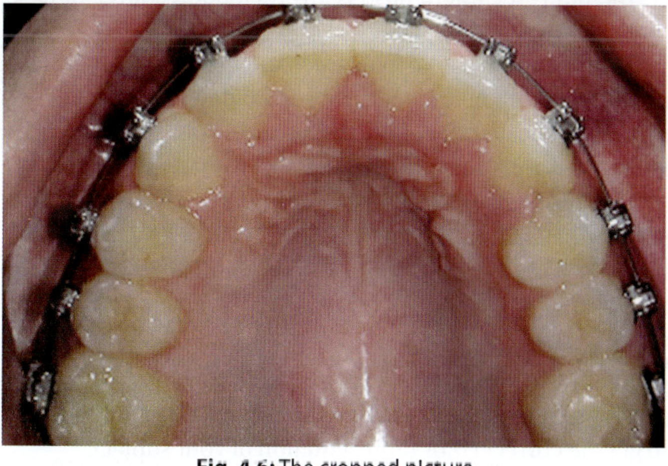

Fig. 4.6: The cropped picture

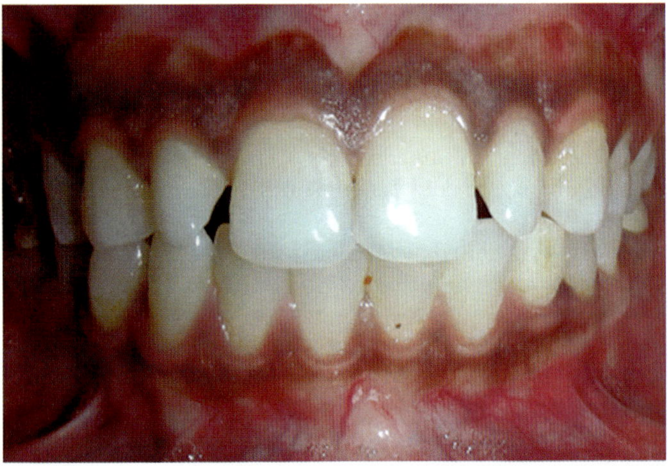

Fig. 4.7: A right-sided flash causes shadows on left side of subject

Conversely, if the flash-subject distance is more than required, it will give a dark picture with incorrect colors.

The built-in camera flash is always a point source of flash and gives distinct shadows.

These shadows serve to distract attention from the subject as in the picture below. One can see shadows on the patient's right side because the flash on camera is on the right of the lens **(Fig. 4.7)**.

This problem is corrected again by increasing the flash-subject distance causing more parallel rays of flash light to fall on the subject **(Fig. 4.8)** and then cropping into the subject **(Fig. 4.9)**.

White Balance Settings in All Cameras

Always set the white balance setting in your camera to Flash, to get the correct color representation of your subject.

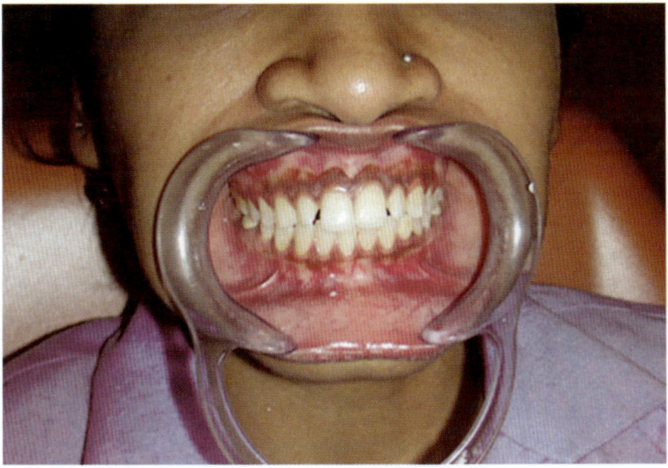

Fig. 4.8: Going away from subject makes light rays parallel and eliminates shadows

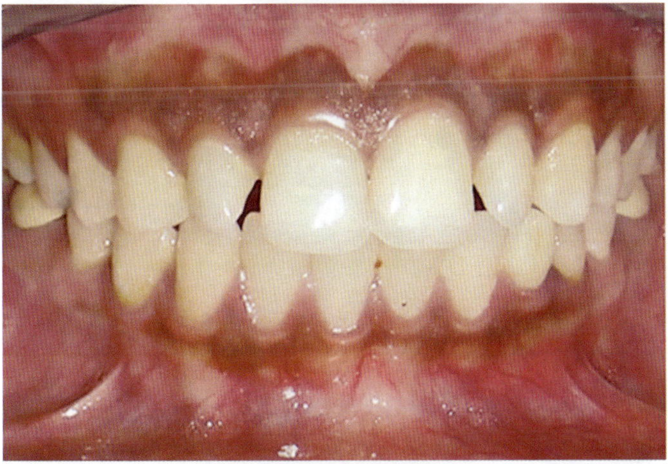

Fig. 4.9: The cropped picture

Use of Ring Flash and Dual Flashes with DSLR Macro Lens

Ring flash surrounds the lens and provides light from all around the lens. The subject tends to get lit from all directions. This eliminates shadows. Ring flashes cost upwards of ₹ 5000 as of date and are mandatory investment to complement an SLR macro-lens. The Sigma EM 140-DG ring flash is an excellent lifetime investment.

Dual flashes provide a two-point source of light and eliminates the shadows that are associated with a single point source of light.

Dual flashes (Nikon R1, R2) **(Fig. 4.10)** can be complemented with diffusers (often part of kit). These flash diffusers soften the light and can give beautifully soft-lit photographs.

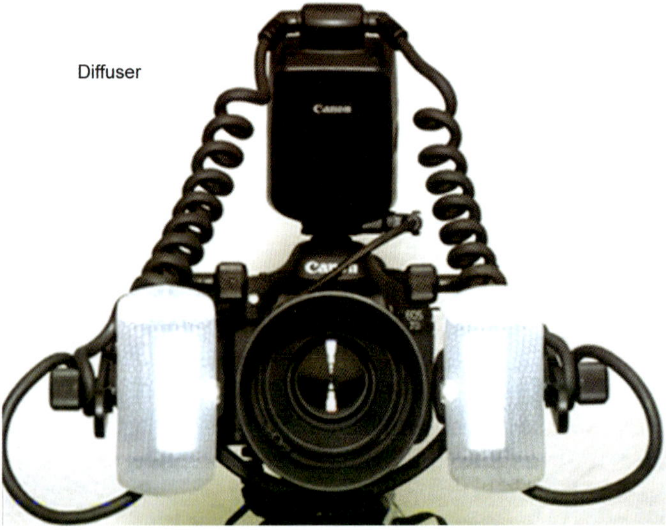

Fig. 4.10: The Canon dual flash

In point and shoot cameras and DSLRs by itself, do keep in mind that shadows are inevitable.

This can be eliminated by two ways.

1. Invert the camera so that the flash throws light from the opposite direction.
2. Move away from the subject so that the light rays fall parallel on the subject thereby eliminating shadows and then crop into the resulting image to frame your subject as required.

USE OF APERTURE CONTROLS

Aperture controls are present in DSLRs and prosumer cameras. They may not be present in compact zoom cameras. Aperture controls can be used for two reasons:

1. To control the amount of light coming in.
2. To alter the sharpness of the picture through the subject's depth (Depth of field).

Aperture Control and Light

Aperture is the hole in the lens through which light enters and reaches the sensor. Much like the iris of the eye. It is commonly referred to as the f-stop.

The f-stops which denote the diameter of the aperture may range from f/2, f/2.8, f/3.2, f/4, f/5.6, f/6.3, f/7.1, f/8, f/9 so on till f/32 or more **(Fig. 4.11)**.

F stands for focal length of the lens involved. For example, if the camera has a 100mm lens, then at f/4 the diameter of the aperture is 100/4 = 25mm.

f/8	=	12.5mm diameter of aperture
f/16	=	6.25mm diameter of aperture

Thus, its seen that as the f-stop increases, the aperture becomes smaller in size.

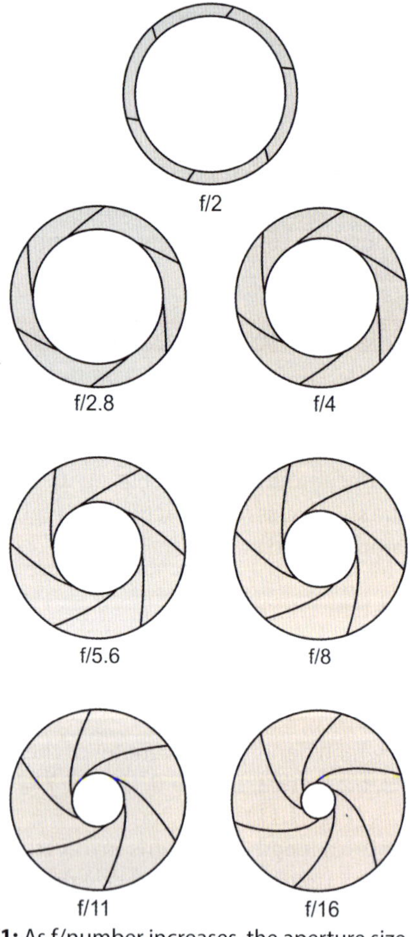

Fig. 4.11: As f/number increases, the aperture size reduces

Consequently, as the f-stop increases, the light entering the camera becomes lesser and therefore the picture becomes darker.

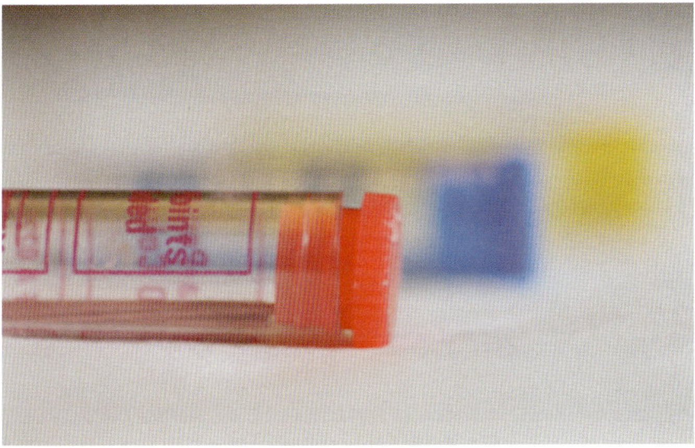

Fig. 4.12: 3 objects at f/3.2

Aperture Control and Depth of Field

As the f-stop increases the amount of sharpness through the subject's depth increases.

For example in **Fig. 4.12**, the focal plane is the red GP box, but a low f/number causes the other GP boxes to be out of focus. Simply by increasing the f/number, the picture in Figure 4.13 now has greater depth of field.

Thus, aperture control can be used to alter the depth of field.

For clinical photography, complemented with an external flash, it is highly recommended to use a high f-stop ranging from f/25–32.

When using manual focus with your DSLR and macro lens, always focus at 1/3rd the depth of the field for excellent sharpness throughout the depth of the image.

For example if taking an intraoral frontal view, focus of the canine to be sharp. Even if the incisors look blurred do not worry, when you click, a high f-stop will ensure that the incisors as well as molars are in focus.

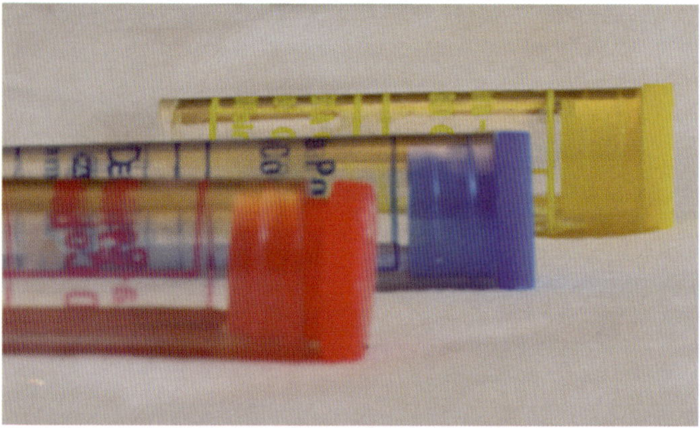

Fig. 4.13: Same subject at f/40

USE OF SHUTTER SPEED CONTROLS IN DSLR AND PROSUMER CAMERAS

Shutter is a part inside the body of the camera that allows the light emerging from the lens to fall on the camera's sensor.

If the shutter has a fast speed, it lets in less amount of light (darker image), but gives a crisp and sharp image.

If the shutter has a slow speed, it lets in more amount of light (brighter image) but the image may be soft or blurred.

Shutter speed can range from a long 30"(30 second exposure) to a slow 8 (1/8 of a second) to a fast 400 (1/400 of a second) to a super-fast 5000 (1/5000 of a second).

Rule of thumb for getting a sharp picture with a handheld camera is that the speed should be 1/focal length of the lens Therefore, while using a 100mm lens, you should use a shutter speed of 1/100 of a sec or faster

When using a slow shutter speed (1/60 and below), there is a chance of blurring of the picture with a hand held camera. In such situations it is mandatory to stabilize the camera with a tripod.

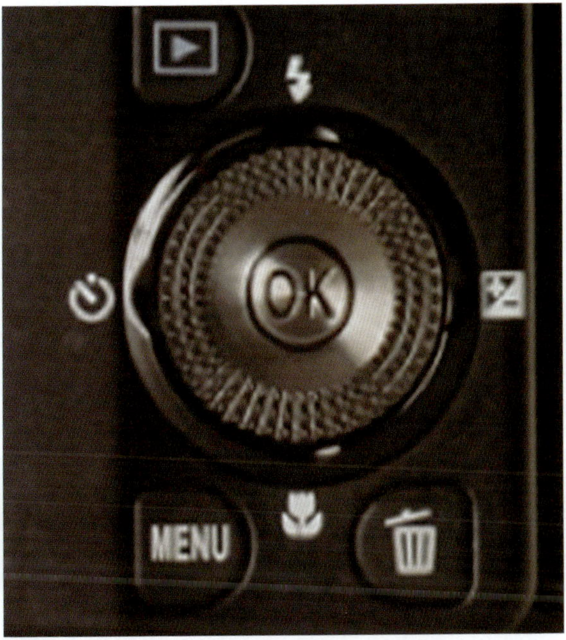

Fig. 4.14: The +/- sign on the right

EXPOSURE COMPENSATION IN ALL CAMERAS

Exposure compensation (Ev) is basically a mechanism to override the camera's automatic exposure mechanism. You can increase or decrease the exposure of an image by upto +5 stops or reduce it upto -5 stops (+2 to -2 in compact cameras).

It is operated by using the +/- sign present in all cameras **(Fig 4.14)**.

In Figure 4.15A, the camera's automatic mechanism interprets the scene as a very bright scene due to the vast patches of snow. Therefore, it underexposes the scene resulting in a dark image.

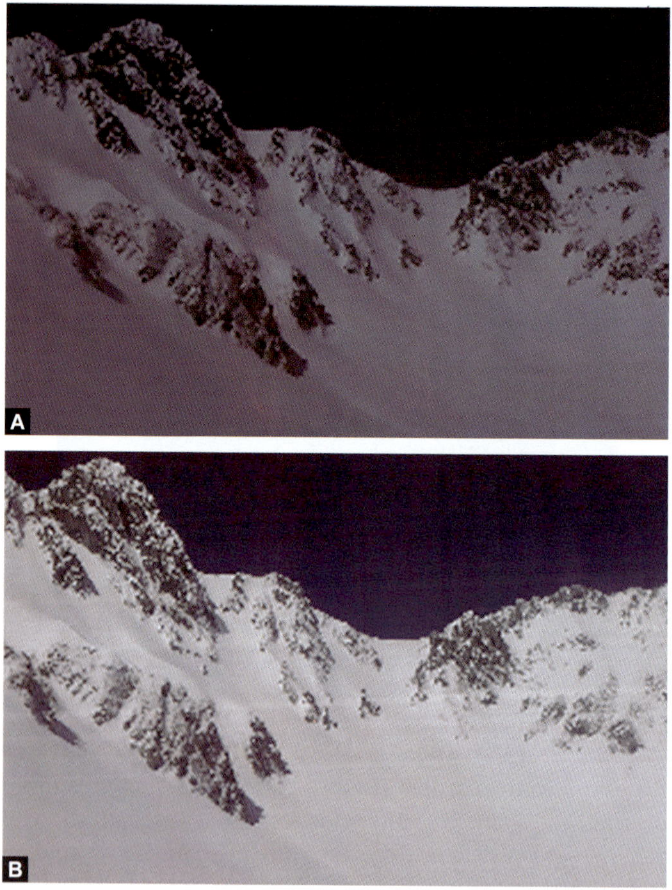

Fig. 4.15 (A and B): The role of exposure compensation

However, one can increase the Ev by +2 stops and obtain an image which looks more like the daylight scene as clicked **(Fig. 4.15B)**.

Exposure compensation can be used to advantage even in the clinical situation.

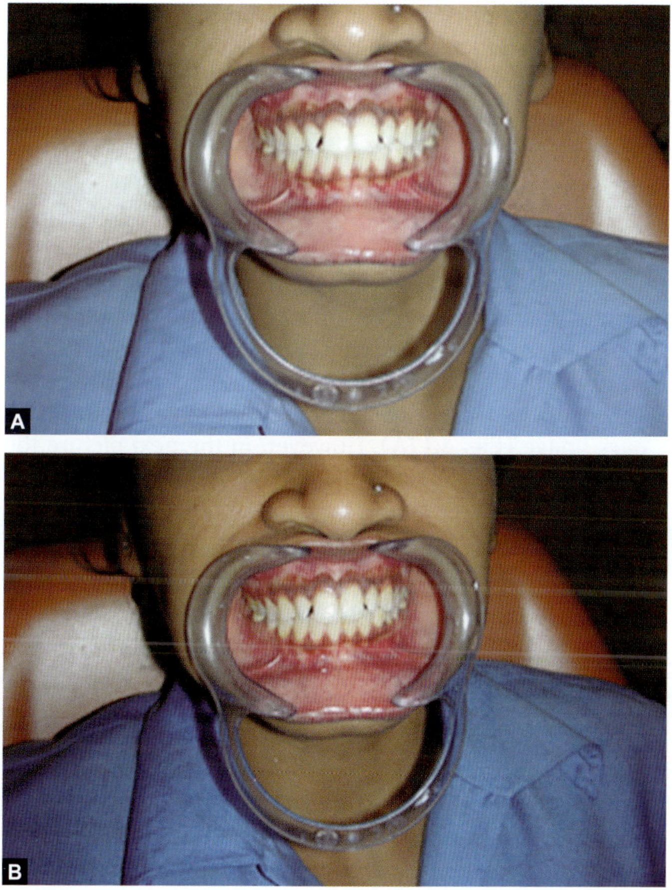

Figs. 4.16 (A and B): Role of exposure compensation in intraoral pictures with compact zoom cameras

In Figure 4.16A, taken with a compact camera, the automatic mechanism has resulted in an over-bright image which has resulted in loss of details in the incisor region of the teeth.

On using an Ev of -1, the overall brightness of the image has been reduced and results in no loss of details **(Fig. 4.16b)**.

ISO CONTROLS IN ALL CAMERAS

International Standards Organization (ISO) represents the sensitivity of the sensor to the available light. ISO is generally available in the range of 100, 200, 320, 400 and so on to upto 6,400 or in advanced cameras even upto 100,000 or more.

Higher you set ISO on the camera, the camera sensor becomes that much more sensitive to light.

The picture of a young boy was taken inside a dark shed. Due to the extremely low ambient light, and at a low ISO of 100, the sensor was not sensitive to the available light and gave a dark image **(Fig. 4.17A)**. However, in the next picture the ISO was increased to 1000. This makes the sensor extremely sensitive to whatever light is available and an image with the right exposure was achieved **(Fig. 4.17B)**.

Always try to use an ISO as low as possible in clinical photography because at higher ISO though the picture becomes brighter it also shows a lot of graininess, technically termed as "noise".

INTERPLAY BETWEEN ISO, APERTURE, SHUTTER SPEED

ISO settings, aperture and shutter speed are three important factors that determine the correct exposure of your subject. If you are getting an incorrect exposure, you can alter any of these three to get the correct exposure.

For a Dark Image to Become Bright

Lack of light is always a challenging situation in photography. You can increase ISO or widen aperture (reduce f-stop) or reduce the shutter speed.

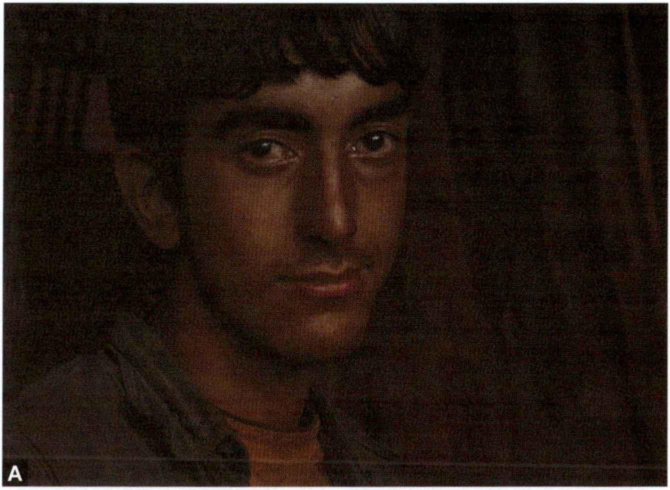

Fig. 4.17A: Low ISO image

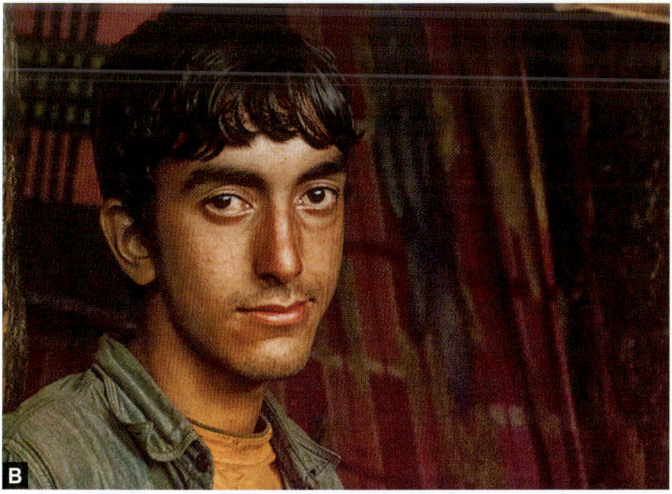

Fig. 4.17B: High ISO image

Reducing shutter speed will either require stable hands or stabilization with tripod.

Increasing ISO will however increase the graininess of the image.

For a Bright Image to Become Dark

Excess of light is always a happy situation to be in photography.

You can reduce the ISO to as less as possible or make the aperture narrower (increase f-stop) or use a faster shutter speed.

BARREL DISTORTION

This problem often arises but escapes unknown when using a point and shoot camera, or a DSLR camera with zoom lens for very close-up shots.

In Figure 4.18A the camera has been held too close to the patient's face while clicking a portrait. This results in a distortion of the subject's face, where the nose (parts closer to the lens) looks bigger than it is. The face too shows some distortion.

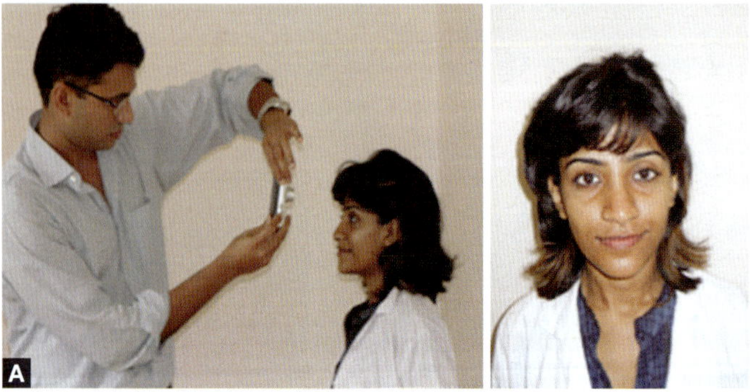

Fig. 4.18A: Zooming too close to patient's face

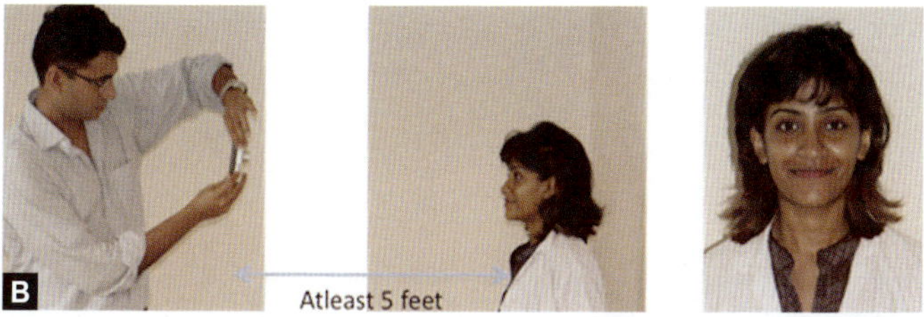

Fig. 4.18B: Not zooming into patient's face (sincere thanks to Dr. Disha Nighot)

This is corrected by taking a portrait snap from at least a 5 feet distance with a zoom lens **(Fig. 4.18B)**.

Macro lenses do not show any barrel distortion even at extremely small subject camera distances

Barrel Distortion in Intraoral Pictures

In Figure 4.19A, the photo was taken with a compact zoom camera. There is distortion of the incisors looking larger and the arch turning inwards posteriorly like a barrel.

Figure 4.19B has been taken with a macro lens. It clearly shows no enlargement of the central incisors due to barrel distortion. The molars are also more visible now.

ACCESSORIES

Accessories are required to maintain isolation of the subject, to make the subject clearly visible on the camera, to enhance the light falling on the subject, to eliminate distracting elements from the frame and to stabilize the camera if need be.

Following accessories are commonly used in clinical photography:

- Retractors - To retract various body parts to isolate the subject, e.g. Lip and cheeks in intraoral photography.
- Contrasters - To eliminate distracting elements from the photograph.

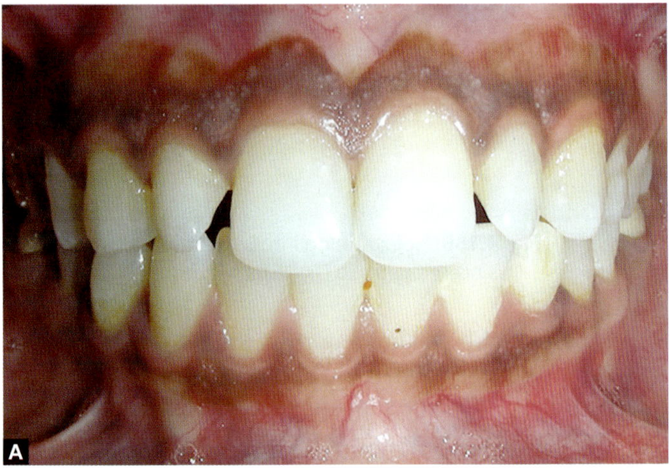

Fig. 4.19A: Barrel distortion with a compact zoom when zoomed close to the teeth

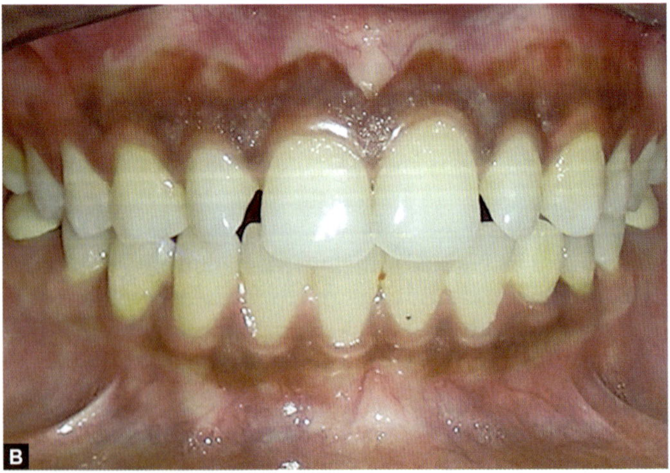

Fig. 4.19B: Not using a high zoom, the distortion is eliminated

- Mirrors - To provide indirect vision when the subject is not directly visible on camera.
- Tripod.
- Non reflective contrast backgrounds.

Retractors

Retractors **(Fig. 4.20A to C)** such as plastic ones are useful for retracting the cheeks while taking intraoral pictures. The single ones help more in retraction than the double ones. All of them can be autoclaved. Metal retractors do not break unlike the plastic ones.

Retractors **(Fig. 4.21A and B)** are useful to keep the lip away when the front teeth need to be photographed or for clicking mirror pictures of the occlusal surfaces.

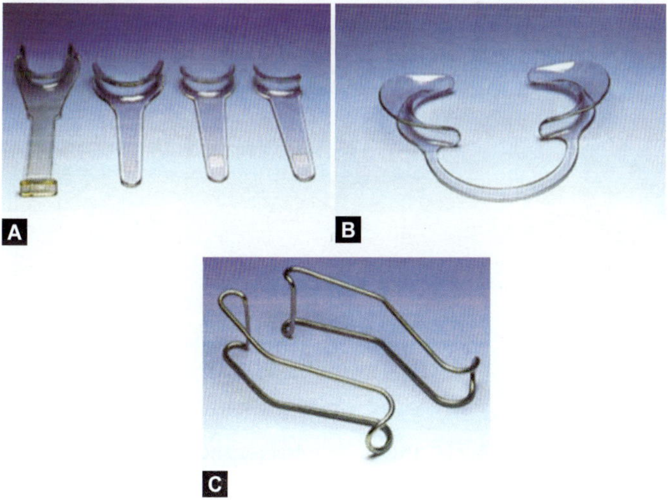

Figs 4.20A to C: Types of cheek retractors

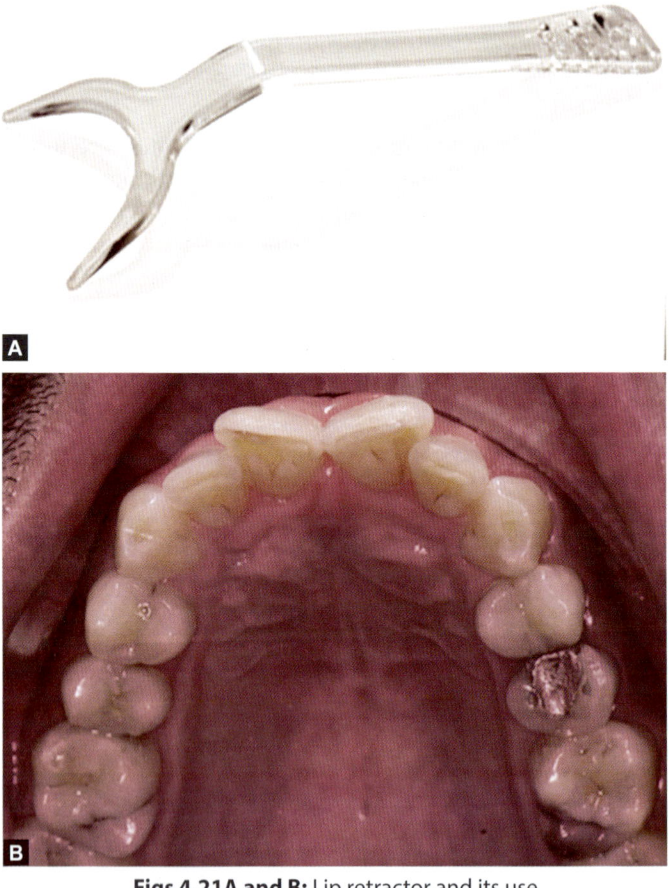

Figs 4.21A and B: Lip retractor and its use

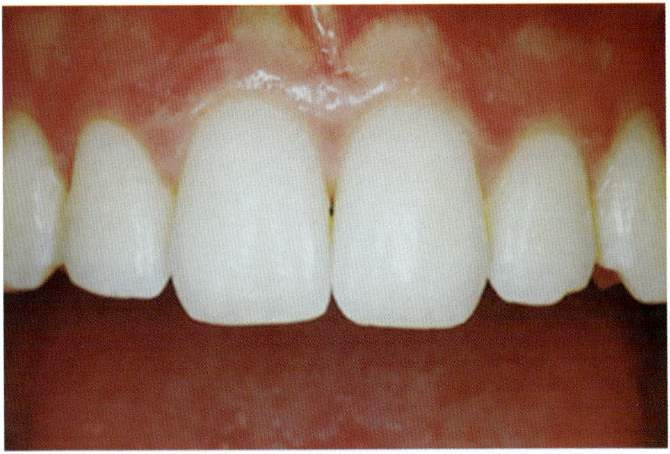

Fig. 4.22: Close-ups with tongue as distraction

Contrasters

In the picture, the tongue in the background is a distracting element that takes attention away from the subject, the front teeth **(Fig. 4.22)**.

Using a contraster, such as ones available from doctorseyes.com is useful in eliminating these distractions. If the patient is holding the retractor, the doctor can hold the contraster himself while clicking the picture. Else, an assistant may be trained to hold the contraster. It should be kept in mind that the contraster should be as far away from the teeth as possible to prevent it from reflecting flash light **(Fig. 4.23)**.

Contrasters enhance the contrast in the incisal portion of the teeth and enable a ceramic laboratory technician to appreciate the incisal translucency and factor for it in the

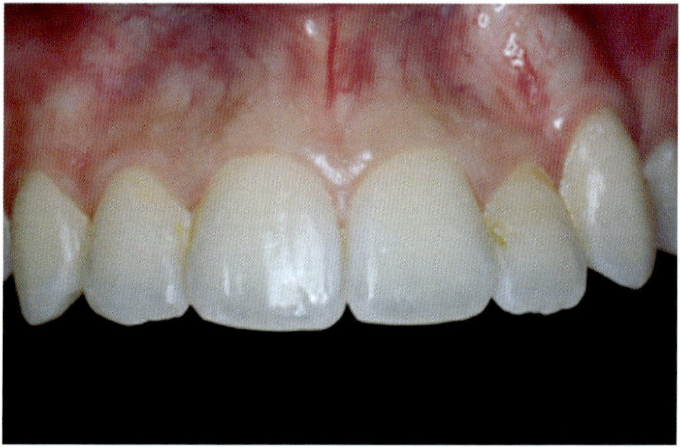

Fig. 4.23: Use of contraster

cosmetic work. The incisal translucency is markedly better in the image with the contraster than without it.

STANDARDISATION FOR CLINICAL PHOTOGRAPHY

Clinical photography skills are developed over a period of time of maintaining discipline.

In each field of dentistry and medicine, the clinical photographs are generally repetitive in nature for each patient. On occasions, a different composition of subject may be required.

For example, in orthodontics, following set **(Figs. 4.24A to E)** of intraoral photographs are mandatory for each patient.

You need to Figure the types of photographs that are to be taken repetitively for all patients in your speciality.

Once you have formulated a list of pictures to be taken, try to standardize the rules for framing each picture.

Ensure that each and every picture you take in the rest of your career as a doctor is taken following the exact same rules and you will have a wonderful collection to be proud of.

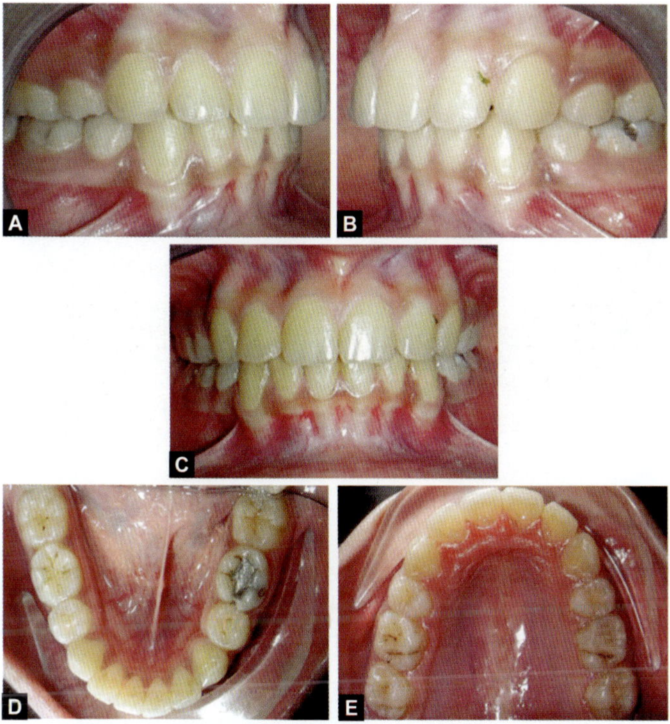

Figs 4.24A to E: Set of standard intraoral photographs

As a guideline, the rules for framing facial and intraoral pictures have been elaborated here. You may take cues and formulate a list of rules for your own pictures.

GENERAL RULES

- Facial photographs can be used either for documentation or for creative uses, such as websites, brochures, etc. For creative pictures, one need not follow rules, but for documentation, one needs to follow 'strict' guidelines.

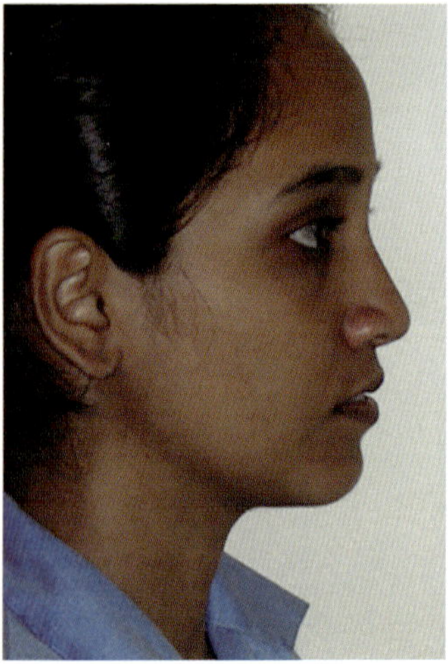

Fig. 4.25: Extraoral profile

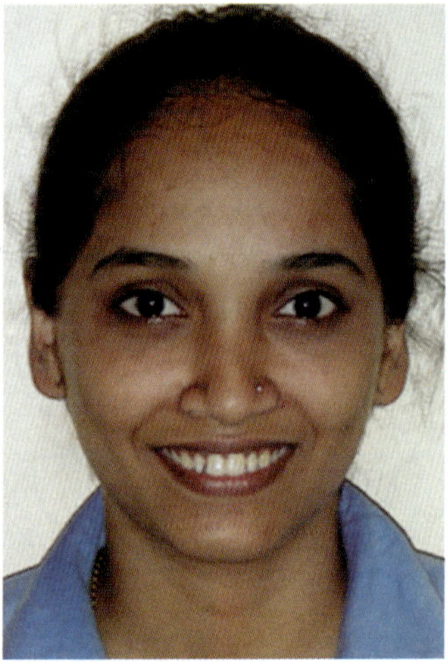

Fig. 4.26: Extraoral frontal

- Use a clean white, off-white, grey, black background with no design patterns for facial portraits. Do not use curtains, the folds and design patterns of which can present huge distractions. Do not use red backdrops. If one is using a green cloth as a backdrop, ensure there are no bloodstains, or any other stains and it is well-ironed without folds.
- Patients are always used to clicking casual portraits. They may not be able to position their head on verbal instructions. One should guide the patient as to head positioning or have an assistant doing the same for documentation portraits.

Rules for Framing a Frontal Portrait

- Head straight not tilted either to left or right.
- Both the ears equally visible, this will ensure no horizontal tilt.

- ❑ The tragion-orbitale-tragion line should be parallel to the floor.
- ❑ The lips should be at rest or in smile as required.
- ❑ Guide the patient should look directly into the lens.
- ❑ Upper frame of the photo should be just above head.
- ❑ Lower frame should be at level of suprasternal notch.

Rules for Framing a Profile Facial Picture

- ❑ Patient should look straight ahead at eye level. Turn head slightly towards camera by 3–5 degrees. Let a slight part of the eyelashes of the opposite eye be visible.
- ❑ Upper edge of frame should be just above the part in the hair.
- ❑ Lower edge at supra-sternal notch level.
- ❑ Left edge just behind the ear.
- ❑ Free space in front of the profile.
- ❑ Face turned to right of frame.
- ❑ Focus on the eye.

Rules for Framing an Oblique Facial Picture

To get consistent turning of the head in oblique facial pictures, try to standardize head position using either of the following techniques:

- ❑ Try to capture the sclera of the left side of the left eye as shown in Figure 4.27.
- ❑ Turn the head till the tip of the nose aligns with the cheek contour.

Rules for Framing an Intraoral Frontal Picture

- ❑ The occlusal plane should be parallel to the sides of the frame.
- ❑ Equal amounts of left and right side of the teeth should be seen.
- ❑ The camera lens should be directed exactly perpendicular to the surface of the front teeth.

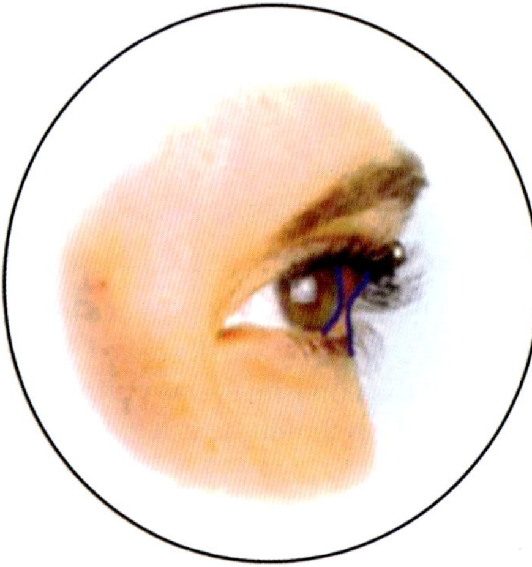

Fig. 4.27: Try to visualize the sclera of opposite eye in oblique views

- Do not direct the camera either from below or from above the occlusal plane.
- All parts of the dental arches should be in sharp focus. Therefore use a high f-stop (22 and above) and focus on the canine region **(Fig. 4.28)**.

Rules for Framing an Intraoral Profile Picture

- Ensure a parallel orientation of the occlusal plane to the borders of the frame.
- Ensure that the distal of the contralateral central incisor is at the anterior border of the frame and the mesial of the second molar is at the posterior border of the frame.
- Ensure that equal amounts of the upper and the lower sulci are seen.
- All teeth should be in focus, so try to focus on the canine premolar region.

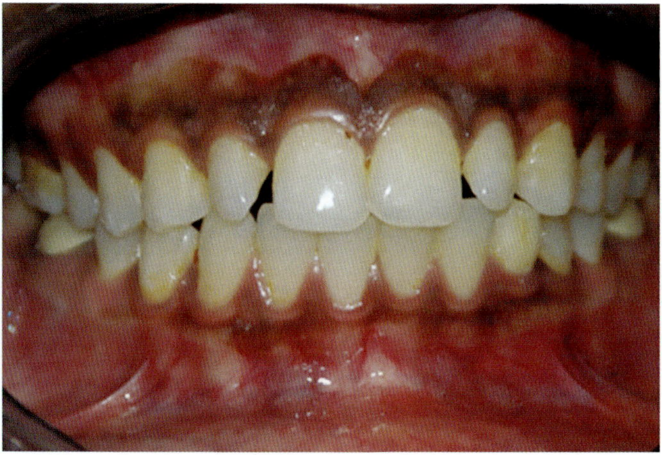

Fig. 4.28: Intraoral frontal

- While using a point and shoot camera, try to keep the flash on the anterior side of the lens to avoid cheek shadows.
- You can use an intra oral mirror to get a more lateral view of the dentition. Use a single cheek retractor on the opposite side of the mirror **(Fig. 4.29)**.

Rules for Framing an Intraoral Occlusal Picture

- Use of an intraoral mirror is mandatory.
- The composition should cover the arch from the distal of second molar to the anterior teeth.
- The indirect view in the mirror should be such that the surface of the teeth are exactly perpendicular to the camera lens.
- Equal space should be present buccal to the molars on both the right and left sides.
- If not using TTL flashes (like Sigma EM 140 DG), since it is difficult to go closer to the plane of the mirror to maintain

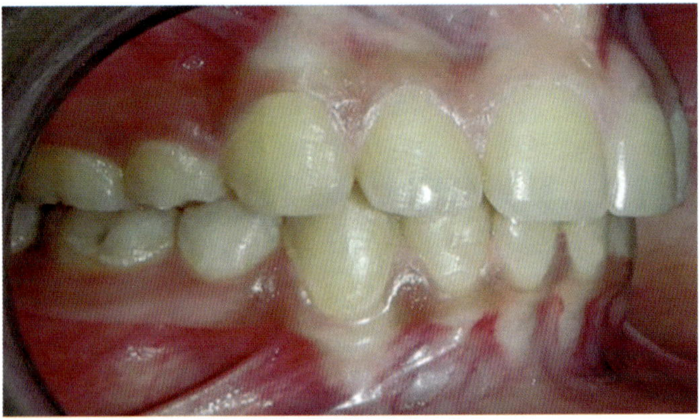

Fig. 4.29: Intraoral lateral

composition, and the consequent loss of flash intensity, it is advisable that the ISO be increased to 400 to get a bright image.

- Fogging of the mirror in the posterior surface can be avoided by blowing air from a distance using the 3-way syringe. Take care to avoid having the nozzle of the syringe in the frame.
- For the lower occlusal photo, the tongue should be out of the frame as far as possible.
- For the upper occlusal photo with a camera flash, stand behind the patient to avoid shadows on the posterior of the frame **(Fig. 4.30A and B)**.

Rules for Framing an Intraoral Anterior Teeth Picture

- The mesial of the canine to the mesial of the contralateral canine should be included. For lower teeth, the extent may be mesial of the first premolars on both sides.
- The teeth should occupy the horizontal middle-thirds of the frame.

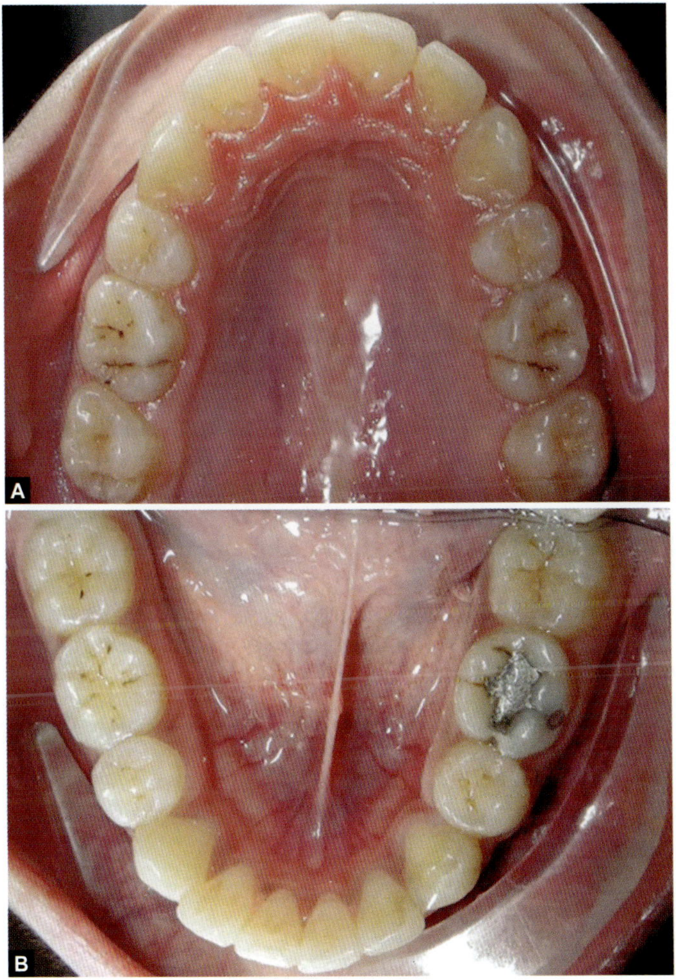

Figs 4.30A and B: Intraoral occlusal

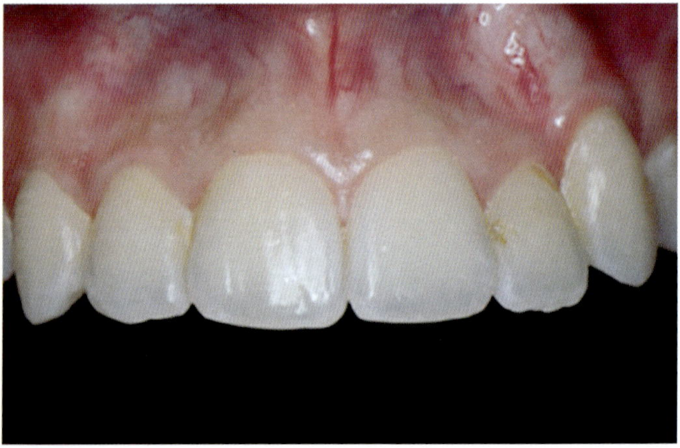

Fig. 4.31: Intraoral anterior closeups

- Contrasters may be used to to eliminate distraction of the tongue.
- Compact zoom cameras may not allow you to focus at such a close distance. So, you may crop the picture according to these guidelines **(Fig. 4.31)**.

TABLETOP PHOTOGRAPHY

Tabletop photography is essential for recording photos of equipment, armamentarium, thesis materials, surgical specimen, etc.

General Rules

Composition

- The object being photographed should be interpretable in three dimensions.
- The long axis of the object should be parallel to the sides of the photo.

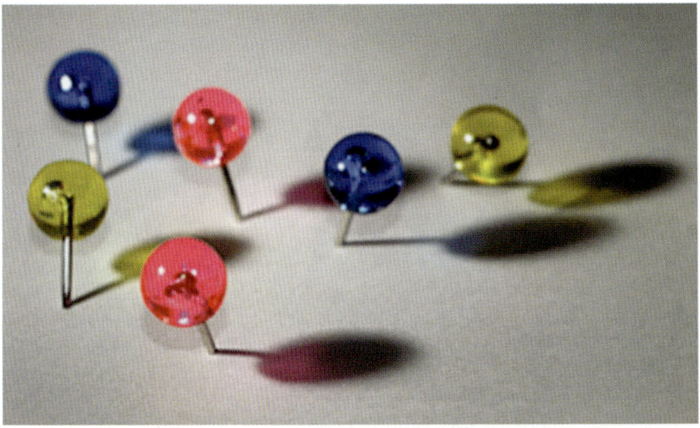

Fig. 4.32: Unacceptable shadows caused by point flashes

- All parts of the object should be in sharp focus (f/11–13 or more) with a narrow aperture setting.
- Since the aperture is narrow, the shutter speed will be slow at ISO 100. Therefore, the camera needs to be mounted on a tripod.

Lighting

1. The object should be well lit with no shadows. A single point of flash can result in shadow **(Fig. 4.32)**.
2. Outdoor daylight with no flash can also give extremely professional results.
3. To eliminate shadows when using daylight **(Fig. 4.33A)**. Keep a white paper on the shadow side **(Fig. 4.33B)**. This reflects light back onto the subject on its shadow side and reduces the intensity of the shadow **(Fig. 4.33C)**.

Background

Always have a neutral colored background against which the object stands out. If it's a light-coloured object, use a dark

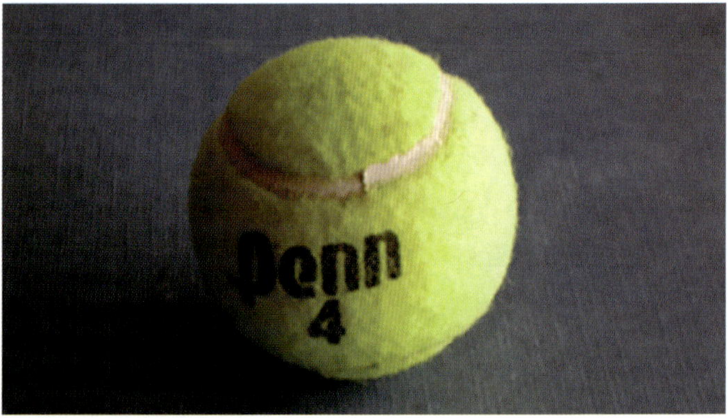

Fig. 4.33A: Shadow caused by daylight

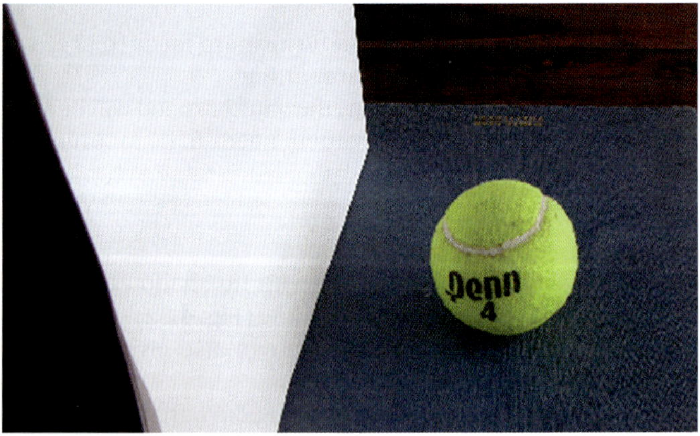

Fig. 4.33B: White paper kept on shadow side

background and vice versa. The background should be clear with no design patterns on it. If you are using a green cloth, then ensure that its clean with no blood stains, etc.

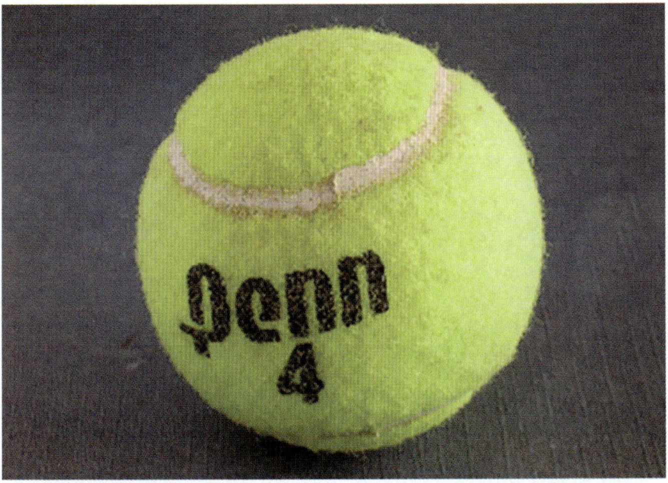

Fig. 4.33C: Reflected light from paper eliminates shadows

PHOTOGRAPHING RADIOGRAPHS

- Switch on the black and white mode of your camera.
- Turn-off all ambient light behind you.
- Mask the excess area on the viewer box around the radiograph with black paper.
- Switch off flash to forced flash off mode. Flash can cause unsightly distracting glares on the radiograph **(Fig. 4.34)**.

SAVING YOUR PHOTOGRAPHS ON COMPUTER

Remember to save your clinical photographs in an organized way on your computer.

Make a folder for every patient and save the images accordingly.

Do give a proper file name that will help in easy recall of the image when needed.

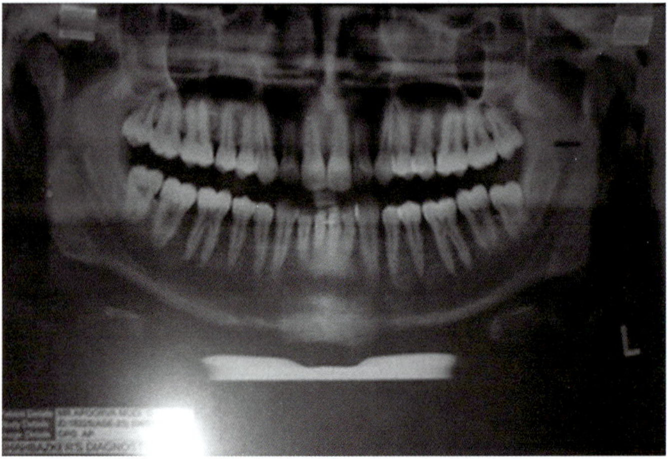

Fig. 4.34: Flash glare can obscure even parts of the radiograph

Do not save the image using the serial number of the photograph as on camera.

COMMON MISTAKES IN DENTAL PHOTOGRAPHY

These are shown in Figures 4.35 to 4.39.

- Incorrect angle due to not using an occlusal mirror **(Fig. 4.35)**.
- Incorrect composition has caused loss of data from the right side of the subject in this frontal view. The occlusal plane is also poorly centred horizontally causing the lower sulcus to be more visible **(Fig. 4.36)**.
- Part of the face and the cheek retractors are distracting elements taking attention away from the subject. Photo needs to be cropped digitally **(Fig. 4.37)**.

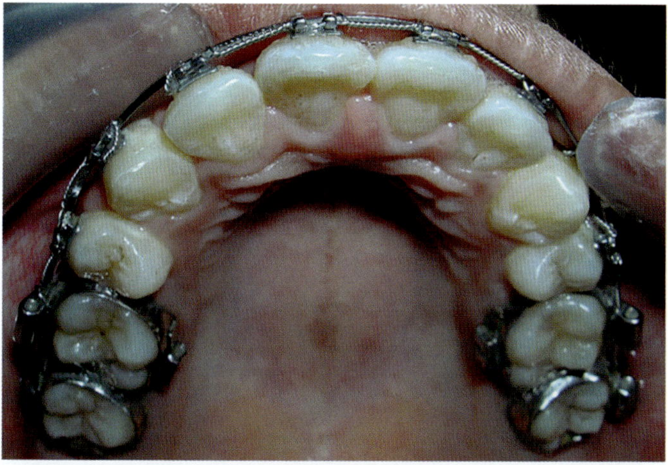

Fig. 4.35

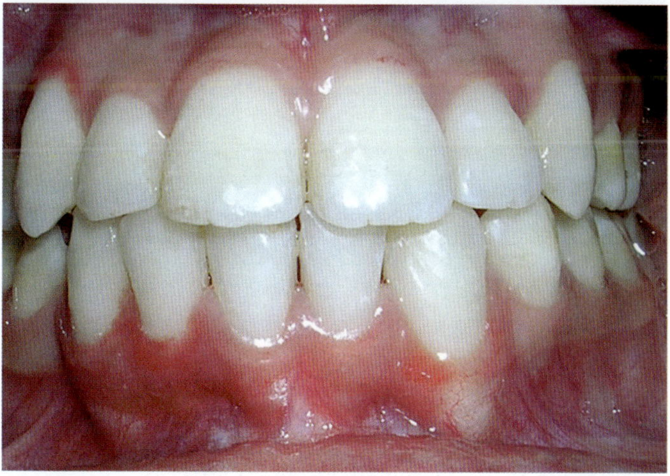

Fig. 4.36

- Blurring due to either unsteady subject or camera shake while clicking **(Fig. 4.38)**.
- Incorrect exposure.

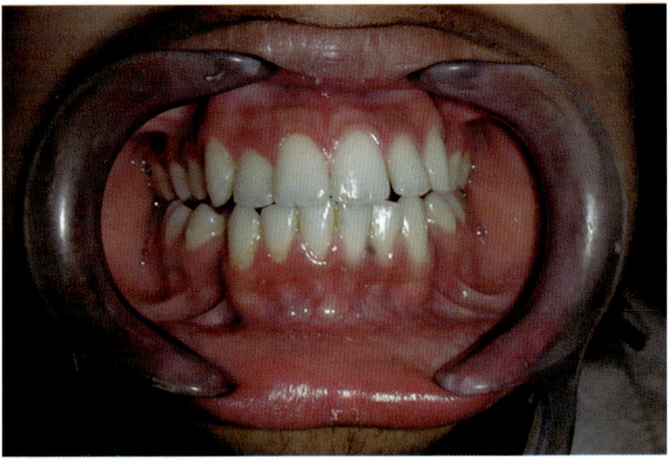

Fig. 4.37

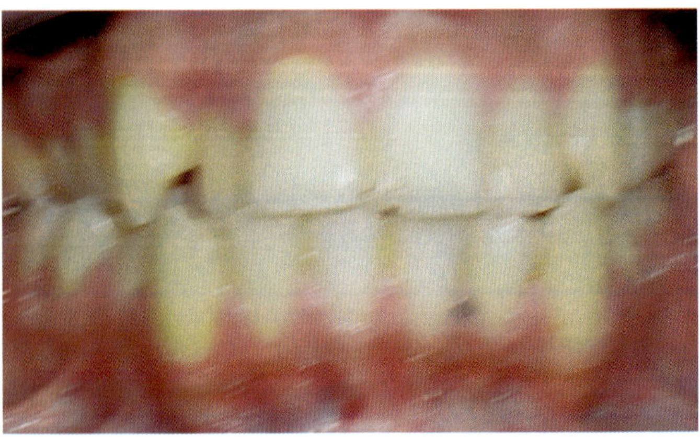

Fig. 4.38

- Severe barrel distortion causing anteriors to look disproportionately larger **(Fig. 4.39)**.

REFERENCE

W.Bengel : Mastering Digital Dental Photography

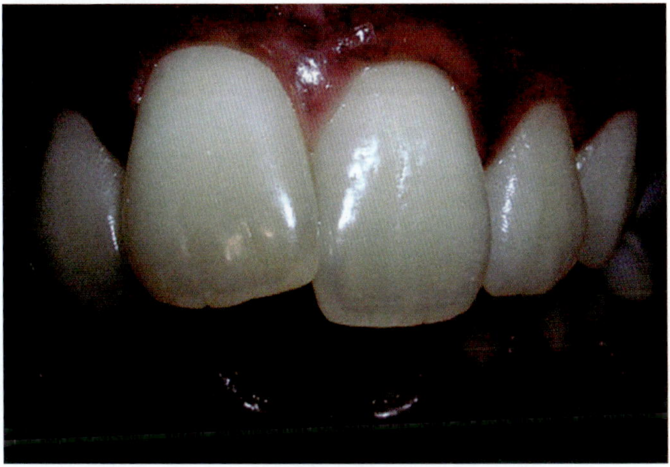

Fig. 4.39

5

Documentation

The Key to Follow-ups

Sudhindra Kulkarni

Outline of Topics Covered

- Need for dental records
- What is documentation?
- What documentation accomplishes?
- Ownership of records
- Components of a patient record
- Financial records
- Written documentation
- Pictorial documentation
- Video documentation
- Types of documentation
- Clinical documentation at doctoral level
- Concluding reminder pointers

NEED FOR DENTAL RECORDS

The need for records and documentation is an obligation and mandatory. As professional of modern medicine/health sciences, we deal with patients and their well-being. At all points in time, the records of the patients under our care is a sacred and needs to be documented and preserved till that point in time as determined by the laws of the land.

WHAT IS DOCUMENTATION?

The information exchanged which can be oral, investigative, therapeutic or instructional between the patient and the professional and allied personnel is a record and is to be documented. This also includes phone records, facsimiles (fax), emails, bills, receipts, image and videos or any other form of recording, such as impressions and patient models.

WHAT DOCUMENTATION ACCOMPLISHES?

- It is an obligation of clinical practice and records the clinician's accountability to his patients and to his professional peers and adherence to the laws of the land.
- It is a basis of continued care and follow-up and recording of changes which happen during treatment continuum.
- It is also a record of the clinician's ability to make informed judgments on patient care in line with evidence-based and good clinical practice.

Figure 5.1 describes all the components of a good clinical document.

The documents must be patient-focused and based on evidence based practice. They should be accurate and maintain confidentiality.

The records are to be made according to practice of their respective profession and organizational policy and procedure.

The documents should help to evaluate professional practice, quality of care, performance reviews and audits and accreditation processes, inspections form legal and governing bodies.

In an interdisciplinary approach, the documents should be shared in a legible manner without any room for mis-information and interpretation.

and/or the institution. This also depends on the contractual guidelines between the clinician and the institution. The law of the land can determine the ownership.

The patients' themselves cannot own, but can always ask for a copy of the records and the clinician/institution is legally bound to give the patients a set of the records.

FINANCIAL RECORDS

The patients financial records should ideally be separate from the clinical sheets and be kept in a separate financial record sheet which is not a part of the case record!

COMPONENTS OF A PATIENT RECORD

The dental record must include each of the following specific components and in detail; these components have to be updated on a continual basis or as and when a change is observed or reported.

- ❑ Medical history.
- ❑ Dental history.
- ❑ Clinical assessment.
- ❑ Diagnosis.
- ❑ Treatment recommendations.
- ❑ Progress notes.
- ❑ Acknowledgement of receipt of notice of privacy practices/ Health Insurance Portability and Accountability Act (HIPAA).
- ❑ Patient consent: general consent and specific consent for specific surgical procedures.

Patient's Assessment

- ❑ Radiographic records
- ❑ Caries risk
- ❑ Informed consent

- ☐ Sedation/General Anesthesia records
- ☐ Trauma records
- ☐ Orthodontic records
- ☐ Consultations/referrals
- ☐ Laboratory orders.

Have to be Updated on a Continual Basis

- ☐ Medical conditions and/or illnesses.
- ☐ Name and, if available, telephone number of primary and specialty medical-care providers.
- ☐ Hospitalizations/surgeries.
- ☐ Anesthetic experiences.
- ☐ Current medications.
- ☐ Allergies/reactions to medications.
- ☐ Other allergies/sensitivities.
- ☐ Immunization status.
- ☐ Review of systems.
- ☐ Family history.
- ☐ Social history of the patient.

Dental History

The dental history should address the following:

- ☐ Chief complaint.
- ☐ Previous dental experience.
- ☐ Date of last dental visit/radiographs.
- ☐ Oral hygiene practices.
- ☐ Fluoride use/exposure history.
- ☐ Dietary habits (including bottle/no-spill training cup use in young children).
- ☐ Oral habits.
- ☐ Sports activities.
- ☐ Previous orofacial trauma.
- ☐ Temporomandibular joint (TMJ) history.
- ☐ Family history of caries.
- ☐ Social development.

Progress Notes

An entry must be made in the patient's record that accurately and objectively summarizes each visit.

Parts of Clinical documentation:

- Written documentation
- Pictorial documentation
- Videos

Types of Documentation:

1. Physical
2. Digital
3. Combination

WRITTEN DOCUMENTATION

Parts of written documentation and their importance in recall and follow-up are listed below.

These are those parts of the patients' record that are discussed between the patient and the doctor. There can be no pictorial description of these parts of the case-record.

These include:

- Chief complaint
- Medical history
- Dental history
- Psychological history
- Family history
- Written and informed consent

Importance of Documenting these Factors

Chief Complaint and History

The change in the complaint and any relief or aggravation of the symptoms of the patient has to be weighed with the chief complaint at the time of presentation. In follow-up and postoperative analysis the patient's perception with chief complaint give an idea about whether we as clinicians have been able to satisfy our patient's needs and solved the problems that the patient had come to us for.

Medical History

The audit of medical history of the patients gives an insight into the changes in the medical profile of the patient and his/her general health. There are medical conditions that influence the outcome of the therapy and/or the long-term prognosis of the carried-out treatment.

In prospective analysis, the continual updating of the medical history and changes in the patient's profile can be related to the changes in the dental status.

For example, a clinically healthy patient who receives a care for a condition A, then over the next 3 years develops a medical condition, such as diabetes and over the further follow-up, if the patient's initial problem worsens, then using appropriate analysis and tools, it may be a possibility to correlate the initial condition to diabetes.

Dental History

The recording of the dental history of the patients and its continual updating is a key tool in clinical management and follow-up, e.g. a patient who has received a clinical care in the form of a crown and bridge today and is recorded as immediate postoperative and reverts back at the fifth postoperative year with secondary caries, proximal bone loss, indicates that, the initial therapy along with factors, such as poor compliance and follow-up have resulted in the patient reporting back with the set of complaints that he/she has today in the current state. This interpretation "today" can be made only if the pretreatment and immediate posttreatment (at the end of the active therapy) records are present.

Family History

The family history and continual updating is necessary to understand not only about the patients' hereditary background, but also about the demographics.

Personal History

The components of the personal history includes a host of environmental factors that influence various clinical outcomes which include: smoking, tobacco chewing, alcohol intake, dietary needs and intake, etc. Most of these factors have a direct bearing not only on the outcome of the clinical condition the patient has presented with, but also the long-term response to care.

For example, a patient who initially reported to be a nonsmoker and over a period of five years, the smoking history is positive, indicates the change in the patient's habit and it is a factor that influences various other conditions. This interpretation can be made only if the initial record is well-documented and recorded.

It is thus imperative that initial recording and documentation is key to evaluating the response to therapy.

PICTORAL DOCUMENTATON

Pictorial documentation is probably the best possible proof that a procedure or a process has been conducted and its outcomes. The pictorial description can be of two types, i.e. photographic images and schematic diagrams.

Photographic Images

This type of documentation is of paramount importance in depicting surgical procedures, esthetic procedures etc. where in a pre-operative and post-operative comparisons are to be made and provide a clear visual change. Certain factors have to be kept in mind while making images, these are:

- The images to be made in a serial order and not retro, i.e. if one has to depict a surgical procedure, then the pre-operative image, followed by incision, then reflection have to made in sequence, it is not that, after the flap is reflected, the flap is replaced and the image of the incision is made.
- All the images have to be made in an DSLR camera, preferably with a macro lens (90–105 mm, f 2.8 and IS).
- Images are better made on manual mode, this keeps the magnification constant.
- All the settings for a particular case have to be same, especially the color tones.
- In case a DSLR is not available, then an amateur camera can be used, but the images made form this tend to be of poor quality and resolution and might not depict the smaller changes!

Schematic Diagrams

These have to be drawn well and need to be scanned at a minimum of 300 dpi. These are an addition to the description of the clinical procedure and images. This usually does not aid in follow-up.

VIDEOS

Videos are a very formidable form of representing data. These are of very high value, especially while describing surgical procedures.

This main drawback of videos is they occupy large space and need to be stored separately.

TYPES OF DOCUMENTATION

Physical

This is the oldest form of documentation and is in a paper, radiograph or chart format and the parameters will have to be entered manually.

This type of documentation is a physical proof and is held legal in the court of law. Certain documents, especially the consent, treatment plan and expenditure at all point of time will have to be in physical form. One can scan a copy and store it in a digital format as a back-up copy.

Even now in India, most of the documentation is in physical format.

Issues

- Storing: Needs space for storage.
- Retrival: difficult and laborious, as one has to sift through reams of data and write it down if they need to analyze a very small set of information, e.g. if one wants to know the sex distribution of the patient's with a particular condition, all the case papers will have to be taken out of the file and then written down and then analyze it.

Digital

This is the best possible format for storing information and aids in retrieval and analysis.

Issues

- Expensive: converting oral or written information to digital, needs lot of time, effort and training. In busy practices and large set-ups, the clinician or staff may not have time to convert all the recorded information into digital format and thus will need a back office (which entails cost).

- The equipment of digital data storage such as servers are expensive and more importantly need constant servicing and change as the technology advances.
- Security: The data has to be locked and saved without any possibility for alteration and manipulations. The software has to have an inbuilt system to record every entry and modification done and by whom. At no point during data retrieval, the patients' identification should be disclosed and should be considered sacrosanct.

CLINICAL DOCUMENTATION AT DOCTORAL LEVEL

At the graduate level of training, the records and documentation play an important role in determining one progress through the learning path. Apart from all the facts of records and documentation mentioned above, as a graduate student documentation is important for the facts listed below:

- Record of all the patients treated: This tells about the experience gained by the candidate through the duration of the course.
- Record of routine cases: This tells about the progress in training from simple to complex cases over the time period of training.
- Record of assisting: In all the branches of medicine and dentistry, "assisting" a senior operator forms a major part of the learning. There will be situations that are very rare and assisting a senior colleague in carrying out procedure in these cases adds valuable experience.
- Recording of work done "under guidance": This category of work is a step preceding independent work. The volume of work done under guidance has to be good enough and this speaks about the "confidence" the faculty has on the operator to graduate to the next level.

- Recording of work done independently: This part of recording and documentation implies that the candidate has gone through all the steps of training, starting at the preclinical level, assisting, performing under supervision and has been found to be competent to let perform the procedures independently. All points the candidates are to keep pictorial/video/paper records of all the work done and which are documented in a format as described by the policy of the respective departments/institutions/specialities and law of the land. All the records need to be countersigned by the respective supervising faculty, only then it is considered valid.
- Records of special cases: There will be situations which are not' routine and the candidate gets a charge to treat them either independently and or under guidance, these cases.
- Documentation for research and audit: As a part of the clinical and training program the doctoral students are to carry out certain research activity and have it published in accomplished journals.

CONCLUDING REMINDER POINTERS

- All data is sacrosanct and has to be guarded.
- Documentation is key to follow-up.
- Long-term follow-up is key to answering clinical therapies and responses and outcomes.
- Follow-up opens doors for appropriate care, course correction and enhancement.

6

Ethical Issues Concerning Your Patient

Sujata Kanhere

Outline of Topics Covered

- Introduction
- Moral theories
- Duties and responsibilities of a doctor
- What are considered as unethical acts?
- Implications of nonethical practice
- The relevance of ethics in current medical practice
- Ethics in the Indian context
- Ethics in the context of a postgraduate student
- The way forward

INTRODUCTION

Healthcare professionals have a responsibility to follow good clinical practices based on ethical principles. Postgraduate students must have adequate knowledge of ethics to analyze and resolve ethical dilemmas pertaining to patient care while keeping within the law.

With recent advances in technology and treatment, it may be increasingly difficult to decide what can be done and what should be done for an individual patient. There is need to be ethical, transparent, reasonable, accountable and remain within the framework of the law, while making such decisions.

This chapter serves to provide a guide to ethics for health-care professionals including postgraduate students, residents, and undergraduate students. Ethics must be applied to all aspects of health including prevention, diagnosis, treatment, palliation, rehabilitation as well as research. Medical ethics is based on certain basic principles and values such as empathy, respect for autonomy of patients, compassion, beneficence, nonmaleficence, justice and accountability.

MORAL THEORIES

These moral theories help in understanding the main moral values governing medical ethics and are essential to deduce whether a proposed course of action is morally acceptable.

- Consequentialism theory: Rightness or wrongness of an action is decided by its consequences.
- Utilitarian Moral theory is a type of consequentialism in which happiness is maximized and harm is minimized.
- Deontology theory states that to be moral is to do one's duty, regardless of the consequences. It involves obeying moral rules.
- In Virtue Ethics theory, an action is right if it is what a virtuous clinician would do in similar circumstances.
- Principles approach: It is a common framework, which recognizes four moral principles in the analysis of medical ethics.

Four Moral Principles that set-out moral duties are:

1. Respect for autonomy: This means that we must respect the patient's right to accept or refuse treatment, take written consent for procedures, verbal consent before examination and remember that patients have a right to have information and make an informed decision.
2. Beneficence. A doctor should act in the best interest of the patient
3. Nonmaleficence: Do no harm to patients.

4. Justice: Ensuring that health resources are distributed such that every patient receives the best treatment, so that justice is done to all. If a certain expertise is not available, refer to colleague with particular expertise or skill so that the patient gets the best treatment.

Moral Duties of Doctors

Doctors have a number of moral duties, such as to preserve life, restore health and prevent disease, to offer treatment that provides overall benefit and minimizes harm, to offer evidence-based management derived from ethically-conducted research. Doctors have to respect autonomy of their patients by respecting their right to decide the treatment options, to obtain appropriately informed voluntary consent, to carry out the above duties fairly and justly with appropriate knowledge, skill and care and act within the framework of national and international law.

Moral Conflicts for Doctors

Medical interventions that are intended in the best interest of patients and with their valid, freely-given consent, with obligations to protect health and respect autonomy, can yet lead to ethical conflict. An important moral issue of best interest arises in children.

Best Interests

A treatment is in the patient's best interests if it confers more clinical benefits than harm. Best interests include taking into consideration age, sex, education, ethnic and cultural background, religious sentiments, physical and emotional needs as well as wishes and feelings of the person. It must also consider the effect of change of circumstances, the risk of harm and the capability including financial status of patient, parents and others to meet the person's needs.

DUTIES AND RESPONSIBILITIES OF A DOCTOR

A. What are the Duties and Responsibilities of a Doctor in India?

- It is the responsibility of a doctor to uphold the honor and dignity of the profession. Nothing should stand between him and his duty to his patient.
- It is the prime duty of the doctor to serve humanity with compassion and respect for human rights, providing competent medical care. He should practice his profession with conscience; reward or financial gain is secondary.
- A doctor should be an upright man, with knowledge, skills and attitude to heal. He should be prompt, confident and diligent in caring for the sick. It is expected that the doctor will be of good character, be patient, modest, sober and conduct himself with propriety in all aspects of his life.
- A doctor should be worthy of the confidence of his patients.
- Every doctor should update his medical knowledge and skills regularly for the benefit of patients. This can be done by being members of professional bodies, taking part in meetings and participating in Continuing Medical Education programs.
- There must be a scientific basis for methods of healing practiced by a doctor. Moreover, it is the moral duty of the doctor to not associate professionally with those who practice otherwise.
- It is the responsibility of every doctor to maintain the medical records of indoor patients for three years from when treatment was started. This should be done in a standard pro forma prescribed by the council.
- Every doctor should ensure highest Quality Assurance in patient care.
- There should be no conflict of interest between the care of the patient and the financial gains of the doctor.

- It is the duty of every doctor to observe the laws of the country regulating the practice of medicine. It is equally important to not assist those who evade the law.

B. What are the Specific Duties of Doctors to their Patients?

- Attending to the sick: Though a physician is not bound to treat each and every person asking his services, he should provide appropriate medical assistance to anyone in urgent need for medical care with responsibility and without any discrimination.

  Every doctor should keep in mind that the well being of his patients is dependent on his skill and attention. He should ensure that no harm is done to his patients. If he is not competent to treat a particular condition, he should refer the patient to an expert in that field.
- Communication and decision making: Doctors must give appropriate information to patients so that they can make informed decisions about their treatment. It is essential to communicate in a way that the patient can understand the information. The patient's decision to accept or reject treatment should be respected. If a patient asks for a second opinion, his request should be respected, keeping the patient's best interest in mind.
- Patience and delicacy: A doctor should be patient and sensitive to deal with delicate issues.
- Privacy and confidentiality: Personal health information of patients must be protected. Confidentiality should be maintained. Information about a patient or his personal life known to the doctor in confidence should never be revealed. It is unprofessional to talk about or comment on or discuss a patient publicly and should be avoided as that may amount to revealing confidential or identifying information. However, as an exception, sometimes a

doctor may have to use such knowledge, to protect a healthy person against a communicable disease or when such revelation is required by the laws of the State.

- Prognosis: The doctor should provide appropriate information about the prognosis of a patient's condition to the patient and his relatives as required in the best interests of the patient and his family. He should neither exaggerate nor minimize the gravity of a patient's condition.
- Attention to the patient: The doctor should not commit an act of negligence leading to deprivation of necessary medical care to the patient.
- Need for consent to be taken by a doctor (respect for autonomy).

Consent

Every individual has a right to choose or decide actions to protect and preserve his health and personal privacy. This is a constitutional right, protected by law. Therefore, any medical examination or treatment without consent is considered an assault on the patient. Hence, consent must be taken before examination or any procedure.

Types of Consent

- Implied consent: Consent presumed to be there. This means that when a patient comes to a doctor for treatment, he has consented for routine examination.
- Expressed consent: Any examination beyond the routine examination requires specific consent. This can be expressed by the patient, e.g. for giving injections, examination of private parts, giving anesthesia or radiological examination. This can be orally or in writing in presence of two witnesses.
- Written informed consent: Refers to written consent given by the patient after being informed of the nature of

the illness, nature of procedure or operation to be done, including alternatives available and consequences and complications. This is the most valid consent legally.

- Blanket consent refers to consent which is taken usually on a printed form at the time of admission authorizing the doctor to undertake treatment. Legally it is no consent.

Informed written consent should be taken before procedures requiring consent from the spouse, parent or guardian in the case of minor, or the patient himself, depending on the situation. However, verbal consent may be enough for examination.

What is a Legally Valid Consent?

It is the consent for medical examination and treatment given by a person himself if older than 12 years of age, conscious and mentally sound, as a written informed consent given in the presence of two witnesses, before the procedure is actually done, given freely, voluntarily and directly, without fear, force or fraud. Consent should be signed by the doctor, patient (or guardian) and two witnesses.

Certain Situations where Consent is needed

- All medicolegal cases–consent is a must for all examination and treatment, after informing the patient that the examination is for legal purposes and may be used in evidence.
- For medical termination of pregnancy (MTP), the patient should be over 18 years of age and herself give consent.
- For sterilization or artificial insemination, consent of both husband and wife is essential.
- Discharge against medical advice can be done only after consent of patient or guardian.

When can Medical Examination or Treatment be Done Without Consent?

- In emergency when the patient is not in any condition to give consent and there is nobody with the patient to give consent but immediate treatment is required to save the life of a patient (Sec 92 IPC). No delay in medical intervention is acceptable for want of consent.
- If there is a chance of spread of infection in the community, examination can be done without consent as in case of epidemics and pandemics, e.g. swine flu.
- Vaccination does not require consent as it is authorized by law.
- In children below 12 years of age, parent or guardian's consent may be taken.

C. What are the Duties of a Doctor in Consultation? Ethics in Clinics and Beyond

- Unnecessary consultations should be avoided. Every consultation should be for the benefit of the patient.
- The doctor should respect the patient's time and observe utmost punctuality for consultations.
- The doctor should have good bedside manners and conduct himself in a professional manner. Permission or verbal consent for examination should be taken. Privacy and confidentiality should be maintained. In case of a female patient, a female attendant or doctor should be present. Care should be taken to maintain privacy specially while teaching students.
- Investigations for reaching a diagnosis should be ordered judiciously and not in a routine manner. In specific situations such as a positive HIV or HBsAg report, it is important not to reveal reports to anyone except the patient.
- When a patient is referred to a specialist by the attending physician, a case summary of the patient should be given to

the specialist. The specialist should in turn, communicate his opinion in writing to the attending physician.

- ❑ When a patient is referred to a doctor for an opinion, he should not take charge of the case. He should not criticize the referring doctor.
- ❑ All prescriptions and receipts should have the doctor's signature and name.
- ❑ Professional fees should be told to the patient before rendering service and not after operation or treatment is being done. Those doctors working for the government or an institution should not take fees from the patient. Fees when charged should be allowed by law and appropriate for the services.

D. What are the Responsibilities of Physicians to each other?

- ❑ A physician should render gratuitous service to all physicians and their immediate family dependants and consider it a privilege.
- ❑ A doctor should refrain from rivalry, insincerity or envy in consultation. There should be no criticism in word or action implying disrespect or impairing the patient's confidence in the doctor in charge or referring doctor.
- ❑ The physician/postgraduate student should treat his teachers with respect and gratitude and his colleagues with respect and dignity.

E. What are the Duties of Physician to the Public and to the Paramedical Profession?

- ❑ Disseminating advice to public: As good citizens, physicians with special training should disseminate advice on public health issues.
- ❑ Notification of diseases: It is imperative for doctors to notify every case of communicable disease under his care

to the concerned public health authorities, in accordance with the laws, rules and regulations.

- Paramedical services: The doctor should recognize that different paramedical services play an important role in treatment of patients and their help and cooperation should be sought, wherever required.

WHAT ARE CONSIDERED AS UNETHICAL ACTS?

Aiding, abetting or committing the following acts shall be considered as unethical:

- Rebates and commission: A doctor shall not give or receive any gift or commission in any form in return for referral or procuring of any patient for medical, surgical or other treatment. He should not enter into contract with patients giving guarantee of successful treatment.
- Secret remedies: A doctor should not prescribe any remedy of which the composition or contents are not known. He should always prescribe drugs which have a proprietary formula and clear name.
- Human rights: A doctor should not participate in or support practices that violate basic human rights.
- Euthanasia/End of life decisions: Practicing euthanasia is unethical conduct in India. The difficult question of withdrawing life support even after brain death, shall be decided only by a team of doctors and not by the treating physician alone, after discussion with and consent of the family.
- Sex determination tests: Sex determination test shall not be undertaken with the intent to terminate the life of a female fetus for nonmedical indications.
- Advertisement: As per the Indian Medical Council (Professional Conduct, Etiquette and Ethics) Regulation

2002, doctors are not permitted to advertize themselves directly as well as indirectly through articles or interviews. However, this restriction does not apply to articles written in the lay press using their own name on matters of public health, hygienic living or even to talks and interviews in other media like radio, TV or internet. Announcement in the press is allowed only when starting practice or changing type of practice, etc, but without photos of the doctor. Also, no sign boards or advertisements showing directions to the clinic are allowed.

- Publication: Doctors shall not include photographs or case reports of his patients which reveal their identity, in any medical or other journal, without permission of the patients.
- Specialization: A doctor who does not hold a special qualification in a field, cannot claim to be specialist.
- Research: Research involving patients or volunteers should only be done, provided ethical considerations are fulfilled, otherwise it is considered as misconduct.

IMPLICATIONS OF NONETHICAL PRACTICE

Although there is no prescribed punishment for unethical practice, but it is considered as professional misconduct and the state medical councils can take action. Warning notice, a written notice issued to a doctor warning him not to repeat his conduct failing which more serious actions will be taken, is given.

Erasure of name from medical register is done in case of serious professional misconduct. This can be temporary as in suspension or permanent which is termed professional death sentence.

THE RELEVANCE OF ETHICS IN CURRENT MEDICAL PRACTICE

Medical practice and medical interventions have changed in many ways. Genetics, stem cell therapy and organ transplants were not possible earlier. Patients are net savvy and can access information easily. Litigations are common. Patients no longer think of a doctor as God. Doctors have to be aware

Do's	Don'ts
1. Be courteous, give complete attention to patients and show empathy	1. Do not argue with the patient or be rude or do any harm to the patient
2. Take permission before examination	2. Do not examine female patient without a female attendant
3. Take informed written consent before procedure or surgery or publishing or research	3. Do not take a blanket consent- it is not legally valid
4. Explain condition of the patient	4. Do not discuss the patient's problem in public.
5. Confidentiality and privacy of a patient should be maintained e.g. in HIV	5. Do not disclose patient's identity.
6. Order only essential investigations	6. Do not order unnecessary investigations
7. Rationalize use of antibiotics	7. Avoid overuse of antibiotics and medications
8. Be transparent about treatment	8. Do not hide important details of treatment from patient
9. Share information with colleagues while managing a patient jointly	9. Do not criticize or blame colleagues in front of patient
10. Refer to an expert in the field, if necessary	10. Do not refuse emergency medical treatment in life threatening situations.

of treatment costs and their implications as well as obligations to the hospital and other authorities. Commercialism and self-promotion is on the rise. Unhealthy competition among health professionals and lack of respect of patient and doctor towards each other are increasing. In this complex environment, ethics and ethical practice become more relevant not only in the interest of the patient but also for the doctor.

ETHICS IN THE INDIAN CONTEXT

India is a vast country with cultural, religious and social diversity. Communication is the key and often lack of communication can create ethical dilemmas. Ethical issues though generally uniform all over the world may have to be dealt with in this context in more regionally sensitive ways which are locally appropriate. Euthanasia is illegal and against the law in India. End of life decisions are difficult to take. Confidentiality, privacy and the importance of consent, need to be emphasized during the training of health care professionals. Medical Council of India has a code of ethics for doctors based on the Geneva Declaration, which must be followed by all allopathic doctors.

ETHICS IN THE CONTEXT OF A POSTGRADUATE STUDENT

Role of Communication

It is important to remember that many of the apparent conflicts in medical ethics arise due to lack of proper communication. When communication breaks down between the health care team and the patient or their relatives or between members of the medical fraternity, it leads to disagreements and strong feelings. These issues can be easily resolved by improving communication.

The Way Forward

As postgraduate students, it may be confusing to conform to different ethical principles and to understand differences between ethical and legal requirements. There may be conflict between their own ethical convictions, the value systems they believe in and what is expected of them. There is a felt need for hands-on training in ethical analysis and decision-making at all levels—undergraduate, postgraduate and by continuing medical education for health-care professionals. The training should focus on improving the doctor's knowledge and developing skills and attitudes needed to deal with these conflicts, to find ethical solutions. When in doubt, consultation with colleagues, authorities, ethics committees and experts in the field is recommended.

CONCLUSION

This is an introduction to the basics of medical ethics in India. The concept of medical ethics, being in the affective domain, needs to be understood and practiced regularly to become internalized during postgraduate training, so that ethical behavior becomes the norm among all health-care professionals.

7

Poster Presentation Guidelines

Sunita Gupta

Outline of Topics Covered

- Introduction
- Advantages of the poster presentation
- Disadvantages of the poster presentation
- How to design a poster?
- Presenting the poster
- Reference Literature

INTRODUCTION

Poster is usually a large printed placard, picture, photograph, notice or an announcement for decoration or to advertise something. It can also be a message or picture which is published on a website or using social media. Posters also provide a major contribution in academic community to promote and explain research work. They are frequently displayed during conferences either as a scientific paper or publication, or as a complement to a talk. Ideally major part of a displayed poster consists of tables, graphs, pictures along with brief text. A comprehensive poster should contain a short title, an introduction, brief description of methodology, results, discussion, references related to the research and last but not the least, acknowledgment to all the assistance and collaboration as well as any financial support received for the research. A scientific poster should be presented with the definitive objective of conveying the information and view to the listener very concisely and clearly. It should be accessible as well as of visual interest for the viewers to notice and take interest in your poster. It should be such that a viewer could fully go through and be able to discern your poster within 5 minutes.

ADVANTAGES OF THE POSTER PRESENTATION

- At meetings so many researches can be shared since many posters can be displayed at one point of time.
- At places where there are infrastructural constraints one can arrange for one huge hall in some convention centers as a session for poster presentation and discussion rather than several separate rooms with audiovisual aids.
- Posters allow viewers to participate in a healthy interactive discussion with no time restraint.
- Interactive two-way information exchange conversation is mutually more beneficial for the audience as well as the presenter.
- It provides a logical and cost effective way of visual communication to the researchers to converse with professionals.
- These meeting sessions can be an expedient place to swap over contact information with potential advisors and employers for further perusal.
- Each and every person can devote time at the poster as per their own field of interest without any constraints.
- Posters are suitable to create awareness quickly as well as for the launch of new products.

- After presentation posters can even be utilized at their own Institution for the students, colleagues, and visitors.

DISADVANTAGES OF THE POSTER PRESENTATION

- Poster designing is the time consuming task as well as requires skills.
- Repetition of the presentation may be required so many times which in turn is a tiring task.
- It is more tedious to carry large posters on the contrary to which oral presentations can easily be stored in various electronic media.
- Few individuals think that oral presentations are more professional as well as formal than poster presentation.

HOW TO DESIGN A POSTER

The Rule of 10s

- On an average, a viewer scrutinizes a poster for 10 seconds from the distance of 10 feet.
- Presenter should be able to introduce the poster in 10 seconds as well as to undertake an interactive discussion and comprehend the useful information to the audience in 10 minutes.

Organizing a Poster

Planning and organization is the foremost step in any graphic design. The very first step is to sort out and arrange the contents of the poster which includes text, images, graphs, charts, logos, etc as it is the most significant and time saving method. Rules and regulations which are provided should be thoroughly read and to be followed while designing a poster.

The very crucial information in regard to this is poster size and poster contents.

Poster Size

The organizing committee of the Conference should clearly provide the dimensions of the poster required. Poster which is larger than required looks unappealing with wrinkled appearance as its size is larger than the slot provided to suspend the poster and also it potentially block the view to adjacent posters. Poster size can be altered and adjusted by the software during poster designing or during printing of the poster.

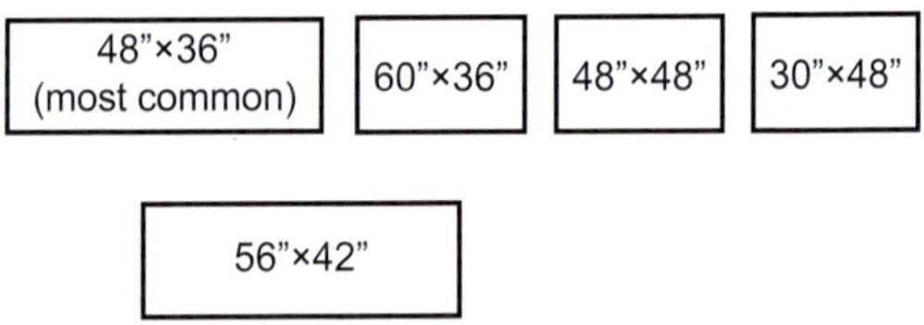

Fig. 7.1: Common poster size

Poster Contents

Typical poster sections are:

- *Title:* A title should be apt, relevant and concise which should attract the viewer's attention.
- *Abstract:* It should be included if it is required.
- *Introduction:* An introduction should be short stating about the topic with brief account of the aim of study and main hypothesis described approximately within 200 words.
- *Objectives/Hypotheses/Aims/Questions:* The testing hypothesis should be described very briefly along with aim and objectives.

- *Materials and Methods:* A defined and concise description of the methodology should be mentioned. Well labeled diagrams, figures and flow charts can be used to illustrate experimental design along with the statistical analyses utilized.
- *Results:* This is always the largest section. Mention whether your experiment procedure actually worked. Results should be clear, self-explanatory described preferably with figures, tables, charts, diagrams. Presentation of data analysis should be qualitative and descriptive strictly pertaining to the hypothesis. If the research is still ongoing then mention about the probable outcomes.
- *Conclusion:* Mention the vital result along with statement about the tested hypothesis whether supported or not. Clearly indicate the importance and relevance of findings and outcome over other previous researches done in the same field along with brief mention about future perspectives.
- *Acknowledgement:* It should be described approximately within 40 words. Acknowledge them who have assisted with their contributions like laboratory assistance, any funding agency, statistical analysis etc. Also include if any conflicts of interest is present.
- *References:* Key references are often required and can be scaled down which are most relevant.
- *Contact Information:* some visitors will want to know more about your research, and you can use this section to provide your e-mail address, your web site address, or perhaps a URL in approximately 20 words.

STEPS IN POSTER PREPARATION

- Everything should appear balanced, appropriate and self explanatory.

- Comprehensive and simple language should be used.
- "Bullet statements" should be used to make points short and clear.

Power point presentation

↓

New file

↓

Blank page

↓

File menu (page set up)

↓

Orientation (portrait / landscape)

↓

Format poster size

↓

Set background color

↓

Choose text box, insert title and all data

Fig. 7.2: Steps in poster preparation

POSTER DESIGN

Storyboarding

Very important aspect is sketching the poster with a pencil and paper. This is called story boarding, and it provides the first, rough visualization of the poster's contents and provides a rough outline of the approximate proportions of space that will be devoted to each section.

The final organizational step is transferring the handwritten storyboard to an electronic dummy or template. A dummy uses filler text and filler images to establish a rough visual layout that can later be filled in with the actual content. By using filler text, one can establish a word limit for each of the sections, write the content of these sections in a word processing software, then quickly and easily transfer each written section into its proper space. Similarly, one can determine the dimensions of figures and photos ahead of time, crop and edit them in the program of choice, and fit them smoothly in place later.

Poster Layout

- ☐ First establish the logical sequence of the material to be incorporated in the poster.
- ☐ Arrange the material into proper sections in a systematic order.
- ☐ Sizes of each content section can vary considerably with each presenter's research content.
- ☐ Arrange material vertically from top left corner to bottom right corner so that it is easier for viewers to read, without having to move back and forth.
- ☐ Material can also be formulated into columns which make it very simple to go through and easily explicable.

Title and Authors with Affiliation: Title should be affirmed maximum in 1-2 lines along with author's details.
Introduction: It should be described approximately within 200 words.

Aim/Objectives: It should be stated within 100 words.

Materials and Methods: It should be described approximately within 200 words.

Results: It should be described approximately within 200 words not including figure captions.

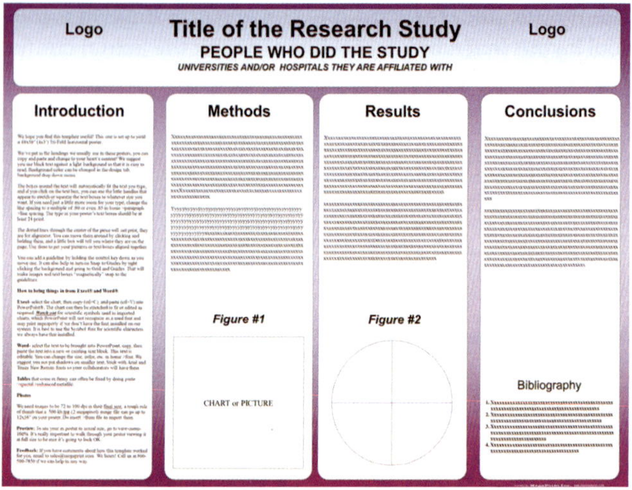

Conclusion: It should also be described approximately within 200 words.

Acknowledgement: It should be provided in less than 50 words in a small font size.

References: 5-10 citations can be mentioned in a small font size.

Font size: Title in 85 pt, Authors details in 50 pt, Sub-headings in 36 pt, Body text in 24 pt, Captions in 18 pt.

Font: Font choice may seem petty in the grand scheme of things, but a good or bad font can really make or break a poster.

Color: Font color must contrast highly with its background such as dark on light background. There is limited legibility with bright colors and complementary color pairs, which strain the eyes. Take into consider those people who may not be able to distinguish between colors. Excessive use of gradients and patterns should be avoided as it does not convey a professional message.

Photos and graphics: Taking photos from the Internet should be avoided. These photos will be low image quality, which prints terribly when blown up on a large poster. Graphs and figures should be saved as PNGs before being imported. PNG is a good file type for images with lots of text and lines, with little risk that they will look pixelated. Pictures can also be saved as TIFFs before being imported. TIFFs tend to produce good quality images when printed on large posters. Large picture for the background or water mark on the poster should be avoided as it can cause serious legibility problems. Shift key should be held at the corner vertices while pulling for resizing graphics. This prevents the image from stretching or becoming distorted.

Softwares for poster designing:

- PowerPoint: It is a popular, easy-to-use option. It is part of Microsoft Office package and is available on the computers.
- Adobe Illustrator, Photoshop and InDesign: It is feature-rich professional software which is good for posters including lots of high-resolution images, but they are more complex and expensive.
- Open Source Alternatives: Open Office is the free alternative to MS Office (Impress is its PowerPoint alternative). Inkscape and Gimp are alternatives to Adobe products.

CHARACTERSTICS OF A GOOD POSTER

- Important information should be readable from about 10 feet away
- Title should be small and draws interest.
- Word count should be of about 300 to 800 words.

- Text should be clear and to the point.
- Bullets, numbering, and headlines should be used which make it easy to read.
- Effective use of graphics, color and fonts should be there.
- Consistent and clean layout should be there.
- It should include acknowledgment, author's name and Institutional affiliation.

SOME USEFUL TIPS FOR POSTER DESIGNING

- Poster should not be too long and densely packed.
- Titles with colons should be avoided.
- Do not add bullets to section headings. The use of a bolded, larger font is sufficient for demarcating sections.
- The width of text boxes should be approximately 40 characters which means on an average, 11 words per line).
- Columns of text longer than 10 sentences should be avoided.
- Wherever possible, lists of sentences should be used rather than blocks of text.
- Italics can be used instead of underlining.
- When using acronyms and numbers within the body of text, scale down the font size by a couple of points.
- Set line spacing of all text to be exactly at 1. Doing this protects the aesthetics if you have used super- or sub-scripted text.
- Dark backgrounds should be avoided.
- Entire poster should be completed on a single platform. Switching from PC to Mac or Mac to PC invites disaster, sometimes in the form of lost image files or garbled graph axes.
- Graphs can be given titles or informative phrases.
- Miniature illustrations can be used to the graphs. Visual additions help attract and inform viewers much more effectively than text alone. Tables benefit from this trick as well.

- ☐ Graphs should not be given colored backgrounds, grid lines, or boxes.
- ☐ Two-dimensional data should not be displayed in 3-D. Three-dimensional graphs look adorable but obscure true difference among bar heights.
- ☐ Details on graphs and photographs should be comfortably viewed from the distance of 6 feet. A common mistake is to assume that axes labels, figure legends, and numbers on axes are somehow exempt from font-size guidelines. The truth is that the majority of viewers want to read only figures.
- ☐ Web graphics should be used with caution. If you're looking for a good generic photograph of something. High resolution photograph should be used so that it doesn't look pixelated (fuzzy) when printed.
- ☐ A thin gray or black border can be used around the photograph to make it more visually appealing.
- ☐ Source of image should be provided which is not yours.
- ☐ Ask somebody to proof your poster, specifically ask them to be super-critical of your citation style.
- ☐ Same font should be used for all of the content section headings. Similarly, all photo and figure captions should use the same font, and all main body text should use the same font.
- ☐ Two complementary fonts should be used wherever possible.
- ☐ Word art should be avoided.

PRESENTING THE POSTER

- ☐ Do not refer to notes when explaining your poster. Speak to your viewers as you explain your poster, don't talk at your poster.
- ☐ Be specific when explaining. Avoid vagueness while explaining the poster.

- ☐ Have on hand, but do not peddle, manuscripts and reprints of your work. If you have space on the mounting board, just pin them up for the taking.

REFERENCE LITERATURE

1. Block, S. 1996. The DOs and DON'Ts of poster presentation. Biophysical Journal 71:3527-3529.
2. Briscoe, M.H. 1996. Preparing Scientific Illustrations: A Guide to Better Posters, Presentations, and Publications, 2nd ed. Springer-Verlag, New York.
3. Day, R.A. 2006. How To Write and Publish a Scientific Paper, 6th ed. Oryx Press, Phoenix.
4. Foulsham, T., and A. Kingstone. 2011. Look at my poster! Active gaze, preference and memory during a poster session. Perception 40:1387-1389.
5. Keegan, D.A., and S.L. Bannister. 2003. Effect of color coordination of attire with poster presentation on poster popularity. Canadian Medical Association Journal 169:1291-1292.
6. Lang, T.A. How to Write, Publish, and Present in the Health Sciences. ACP Press.
7. Matthews, J.R., J.M. Bowen, and R.W. Matthews. 1996. Successful Science Writing: A Step-by-Step Guide for the Biological and Medical Sciences. Cambridge University Press, Cambridge.
8. Pechenik, J.A. 2009. A Short Guide to Writing about Biology, 7th edition. Longman, New York.
9. Rigden, C. 1999. 'The eye of the beholder'- designing for color-blind users. British Telecommunications Engineering 17:2-6.
10. Tufte, E.R. 1983. The Visual Display of Quantitative Information. Graphics Press, Connecticut

11. Wolcott, T.G. 1997. Mortal sins in poster presentations or, How to give the poster no one remembers. Newsletter of the Society for Integrative and Comparative Biology Fall: 10-11.
12. Woolsey, J. D. 1989. Combating poster fatigue: how to use visual grammar and analysis to effect better visual communications. Trends in Neurosciences 12:325-332.

8

The Art of Scientific Writing

Sabita M Ram

Outline of Topics Covered

- Introduction
- Referencing for citing
- Different forms of citing
- Reasons for referencing
- Vancouver's system
- Citing different sources using Vancouver system

INTRODUCTION

"Science is the mistress of modern world." We, medical professionals, are surrounded by a mass of information. It is essential that we acquire relevant, accurate and up-to-date knowledge in our subject area. We gather information, which are transferable skills that we need in the future, to prepare seminars, discussions, research projects, etc. Literature review and process of compiling a comprehensive list of reference that one has consulted in one's writing plays an important role in the research process. An incomplete and inaccurate list of reference reflects on the quality of work and may devalue the impact.

REFERENCING FOR CITING

It is a standardized method of acknowledging source of information and ideas one has used in one's writing in a way that uniquely identifies the source.

Different Forms of Citing

- Reference list: It has all the items one has directly or indirectly cited in the text.
- Bibliography: It contains list of additional works to which one has not directly made reference to, but has helped one construct the essay.

Sources of Information

Formal	*Informal*
Dictionaries	Discussion list
Directories	Websites
Encyclopaedias	Grey literature
Books	
Journals	

Reasons for Referencing

Important reasons for referencing are to:

- Give proper credit to other people's works and ideas (taking other person's thoughts, words, judgments, ideas, etc.), as one's own, without any indication that they are those of another person which constitutes plagiarism.
- Show that one has consulted widely, recognizing and acknowledging the relevant debate, arguments and practice in a given field.

- Substantiate any statement that one makes in a research.
- Signpost other to related works and prior publications.
- Enable others to check the evidence and accuracy of one's information and to consult texts which one has found relevant and useful.
- Enable one to go back to review the sources of his/her information.

Elements for Referencing

Item	*House Style*	*Choice of referencing*
Books	Underlining	Vancouver
Journals	Highlighting	Harvard
Newspapers	Quotation	MHRA
Electronic journals		MLA
		APA

MHRA, Modern Humanities Research Association; MLA , Modern Language Association of America; APA, American Psychological Asssociation

Vancouver's System

It is commonly used for medical referencing. It is also known as numeric approach or citation sequence approach.

System was devised when a small group of general medical journal editors met informally in Vancouver, British Columbia in 1978 to establish guideline for the format of manuscripts submitted to their journals. The group came to be known as the Vancouver group.

Group expanded and evolved into the International Committee of Medical Journal Editors (ICMJE), which meets annually. The ICMJE has produced multiple editions of the "Uniform Requirements for Manuscripts submitted to Biomedical Journals" (first published in 1979). It also discusses issue relating to ethical principals as applied to publication in biomedical journals.

Guidelines

1) References are indentified by Arabic numbers, written as superscripts or enclosed in square bracket.
2) It is important to be consistent when one is referencing.
3) If referencing list is continuous, it is joined by a hyphen. For example, 2-5.
4) If list is separated, use commas without spaces. These are used in multiple citations. For example, 2,3,4,5.
5) Number sequence will follow the essay as and when it appears.
6) Reference number should be same even if the reference is repeated.
7) The placement of citation numbers within text should be carefully considered, for example a particular reference may be relevant to only part of a sentence. As a general rule, reference numbers should be placed outside full-stops and commas, inside colons and semicolons; however, this may vary according to the requirements of a particular journal.
8) If only a part of the sentence is referred, number should be put at end of the piece of reference.

Examples

- Reference in brackets: The cracked tooth syndrome is defined as the incomplete fracture of the nature crown of a premolar or molar tooth. [3]
- Reference as superscript: Gibbs[4] in 1954 was the first author to describe an incomplete fracture in the dental literature, using the term *cuspul fracture odantalgia.*

CITING DIFFERENT SOURCES USING VANCOUVER SYSTEM

Citing a Book

The essential details required are listed below in the order:

Name(s) of author, editor(s) or compilers

Rules

- Where there are six or fewer authors, all authors must be listed.
- Where there are more than six authors, only first six are listed and "et al" mentioned after that.
- A comma and one space are put between each name. There must be a full stop after the name of the last author.
- No punctuation to be used between initials.
- Name of the author is self-explanatory.
- If author's name is not available, editor's name (if mentioned) to be written.
- The word editor or editor(s) should follow the list of editors. Full list has to be written in bibliography irrespective of the number of authors/ editors.

Examples

- Name of the author: Shore NA.
- Name of the editors: Storer R, Skinner EW, editors.
- More than six editors: Fauci AS, Braunwald W, Isselbacher KJ, Wilson JD, Martin JB, Kasper DL, et al, editors.

Format

- Surname (one space) initial/s.
- Full-stop after the last name followed by one space.

Title of publication

Rules

- Do not use italics or underlining.

- ☐ Only the first word of journal article or book titles (words that normally begin with capital letter) is capitalized.

Format
Title (fullstop, one space)

Example
Shore NA. Temporomandibular joint dysfunction and occlusal equilibration.

Edition

Rules
- ☐ Not mentioned if it is first edition
- ☐ Abbreviated as 'ed'

Format
Edition number (full-stop, one space)

Example
Shore NA. Temporomandibular joint dysfunction and occlusal equilibration. 2nd ed.

Place of Publication

Rules
- ☐ If the publishers are located in more than one city, cite the name of the city that is printed first.
- ☐ Write the place name in full.
- ☐ If the place is not well known, add a comma, one space and the state or country for clarification.

Format
Place of publication (colon, one space)

Example
Shore NA. Temporomandibular joint dysfunction and occlusal equilibration. 2nd ed. Philadelphia:

Publisher

Rule
Publisher name should be printed in full.

Format
Publisher (semicolon, one space)

Example
Shore NA. Temporomandibular joint dysfunction and occlusal equilibration. 2nd ed. Philadelphia: JB Lipincott;

Year

Format
Year (full-stop, add one space if page number follows)

Example
Shore NA. Temporomandibular joint dysfunction and occulsal equilibration. 2nd ed. Philadelphia: JB Lipincott; 1976.

Page number (if applicable)

Rules
- Abbreviated as "p."
- Do not repeat digits unnecessarily.

Format
p (full-stop, one space) page numbers (full-stop)

Example
Shore NA. Temporomandibular joint dysfunction and occlusal equilibraton. 2nd ed. Philadelphia: JB Lipincott; 1976. p. 112–9.

Series title and individual volume, if any

Rules
- Put in brackets
- Abbreviate the word volume to "vol"

Format
(Series title (semicolon, one space) vol (one space) volume number) full-stop outside the bracket.

Example
Bennett GL, Horur R. Iodination of chemokines for use in receptor binding analysis. New York : Academic press; 1997. p.134-48. (Methods in enzymology; vol 288).

Citing Dictionary and Similar References

Contents

- ☐ Title of the book
- ☐ Edition
- ☐ Place of publication
- ☐ Publisher
- ☐ Year
- ☐ Definition looked up
- ☐ Page number.

Format is same as that of citing a book.

Example

Stedman's medical dictionary. 26th ed. Baltimore: Williams & Wilkins; 1995. Apraxia; p. 119-20.
(Definition looked up- in this case "apraxia")

Chapter or Part of a Book to Which a Number of Authors have Contributed

Contents

1) Name of the authors
2) Name of the chapter/ part of the book
3) Name of the editors
4) Title of the book
5) Edition

6) Place of publication
7) Publisher
8) Year
9) Page number.

Format

It is same as that of citing a book.

Example

Porter RJ, Meldrum BS. Anti epileptic drug. In: Katzung BG, editor. Basic and clinical pharmacology. 6th ed. Norwalk: Appleton and Lange; 1995. p. 361-80.

Citing a Journal Article

The essential details (in order) are mentioned below:

Name(s) of author(s) of the article

See step 1 of citing of book for full details

Example
Kakade D, Vadgaonkar P, Gupta A.

Title of the article

Format is same as title of publication. See step two of citing of book for full details.
Example: Kakade D, Vadgaonkar P, Gupta A. Obturator for a maxillectomy patient.

Title of journal

Rules

- Abbreviate the title as per the list in the most recent issue of Index Medicus.

- No punctuation is used in the abbreviated journal name.

Format

- Abbreviated journal title (one space).

Example

Kakade D, Vadgaonkar P, Gupta A. Obturator for a maxillectomy patient. JIDA.

Year (and month/day if necessary) of publication

Rules

- Abbreviate the month to the first three letters.
- If the journal has continuous page numbering through volume, the month/day and issue information can be omitted.
- If months are available mention them with no space separating them.

Format

- Year (semicolon, no space) or year (one space) month (one space) day (semicolon, no space).

Example

Kakade D, Vadgaonkar P, Gupta A. Obturator for a maxillectomy patient. JIDA.1998;

Volume Number (and issue/part if necessary)

Rules

- Issue number omitted for journals with continuous numbering through volumes.

Format

Volume number (no space) issue number in brackets (colon, no space) or volume number (colon, no space)

Example

Kakade D, Vadgaonkar P, Gupta A. Obturator for a maxillectomy patient. JIDA. 1998; 69:

Page numbers

Rules

Do not repeat digits unnecessarily.

Format

Page numbers (full-stop)

Example

- Kakade D, Vadgaonkar P, Gupta A. Obturator for a maxillectomy patient JIDA.1998; 69:188-90.
- Noncontinuous page numbers : 1996 Jun 1; 12(5):127-33.
- Continuous page numbers : 1996; 12:127-33.

Citing a Newspaper

Rules

- First letter of the words are capitalized
- Section of the newspaper to be mentioned where the article appears.
- Section abbreviated as "sect".
- Column number to be written and is abbreviated as "col". This has to be put in brackets.

Format

- Same as citing a book.

Contents

- Author, if given
- Title of the article
- Name of news paper
- Date of edition (year month day); section if applicable
- Series, if applicable
- Page number
- Column number in brackets.

Example:

Calcium for living bones. The Times of India. 2004 Jan 25: Sect. Times wellness: 3(col.2).

Citing Pamphlet

Rules

Pamphlet should be written in square brackets.

Format

Similar to citing a book.

Example

Colgate total plax. Product Information [Pamphlet]. Colgate - Palmolive (India ltd); 2003.

Citing Internet and other Sources

Rules

Source may be subjected to alteration. It is important to acknowledge the date at which the information was accessed. This is particularly true for web sites that may disappear or permitted to changes and CD-ROMS, which may be updated during the year.

Format for citing a journal on Internet

- Similar to citing a journal.
- Abbreviated title of electronic journal to be written followed by "serial online" in square brackets.
- URL mentioned.
- Number of screens mentioned in square brackets or pages.
- Available from URL address.
- Accessed month in full, day of month and year.

Example

Morse SS. Factors in the emergence of infectious disease. Emerg Infect Dis [serial online] 1995; 310:1387-90. Available from: URL:http://www/cdc/gov/ncidoc/EID/eid.htm. Accessed December 25,1999.

Citing CD-ROM

Rules

- Similar to citing a book.
- Book on CD-ROM to be mentioned in brackets.

Example

The Oxford English Dictionary [book on CD-ROM]. 2nd edition. New York, NY: Oxford University Press; 1992.

Note: Certain sections of the examples have been highlighted only for illustration. Do not use underlining while citing.

9

The Art of Dissertation Writing

Aditya Mitra

Outline of Topics Covered

- Introduction
- Now the question arises, how to choose a dissertation topic?
- How to select a dissertation topic?
- Some Special Considerations

INTRODUCTION

A thesis or dissertation is a document submitted in support of candidature for an academic degree or professional qualification presenting the author's research and findings.

A master's degree thesis is more closely related to a research paper that you would have completed during college. You are expected to use the research of others and provide your own analysis on your discoveries. It demonstrates your level of critical and analytical thinking and defines the subject that you are most interested in pursuing within your field.

The primary purpose of a thesis or dissertation is to train the student in the processes of scholarly research and writing under the direction of members of faculty. After the student has passed and the work is published, it serves as a contribution to human knowledge, useful to other scholars and perhaps even to a more general audience.

Dissertation is partial fulfilment of requirements in achieving a master degree. It is not everything, but it is an important step. If you have a good dissertation, you have already impressed your internal and external examiner and moderator. You have scored a mark in job interviews or further studies in India or abroad. Even if you will be in private practice, your juniors will admire your dissertation and you never know you can be in academics even 10–15 years later.

Now the question arise, how to choose a dissertation topic:

- Ideally it should be an original study; if you opted for an easy way out, please do not replicate an existing study, change the variables or the factors in the study.
- Before finalizing the topic, please think about clinical implications.
- If it is an *in vitro* study, can it be replicated *in vivo*?
- Or, a theoretical question-what is the clinical implication?
- It should ultimately benefit the patients and practising dental surgeons both.

HOW TO SELECT A TOPIC

- Pick such a topic, which is interesting to you as well as to others.
- While you think about your subject, think about the top 3 questions (related to your subject) which always come to your mind and have drawn your interest.
- Search articles in different journals related to that topic and questions. Find articles which are dealing with relatively new research, less work has been done on it but which provoke interest. Newer topic will give you more scope for invention of new facts related to that topic.
- If you have done any hands on or coursework in your speciality during your undergraduate level or afterward which attracted you, then you may try to find a topic related to that.

- ❑ After choosing a topic, please evaluate its importance in relation to ongoing research or unsolved question, its significance in theory as well as in practical.
- ❑ If you have selected a topic on which no work / research had done before, then please try to find the reason why no work had done before on that topic. May be there are some difficulties present in the study procedure, which prevents the researchers to do study on it. If you select the topic without any investigation, then later on you may face difficulties in the midway of your study.
- ❑ During choosing a topic for dissertation, please work with your guide, consult with him/her, take his/her advice; the help and ideas are invaluable.
- ❑ After choosing a topic:
    - Look for the materials you require.
    - The instruments which you need to use.
    - Then think and search about the availability and cost of the materials.
    - The instruments are available or not.
    - If the instrument is available in any institution - then find that institution will allow you to use that instrument/or not.
    - Find out the actual procedure to get the permission of the use of the instrument in any other institution.
    - And if it is not readily available, then think if you can use it in any clinic?.
    - Find out whether you can afford the total cost of the procedure, if "yes" then only proceed, if "not" then leave the topic; search for a new one.
- ❑ If you are thinking of studying on new materials, it is good but always remember, sometimes it is difficult if the mechanism of action or role of each constituents are not known properly.
- ❑ After choosing a topic, think about the whole procedure, please think, whether the total procedure can be

completed within 18–21 months (6 months for selection and pilot study + 12 months for the work done and study procedure + 3 months for summing-up the results, final analysis and write-up); if "yes" only then proceed, if "not" then don't run after it. Earlier 'time limit' was an important thing in post-graduation dissertation process—you had to complete the whole work and submit it on time.

- Please think, whether good data can be collected from your study or not, because sometimes it happens that the topic is interesting but the collection of data is difficult and impossible within the circumstances, in that cases you can't analyze your study.
- Use a systematic approach–organize notes and references from the very beginning. When you are selecting an article, always maintain proper references, so that during the actual work it will make things easy.
- Please find whether anyone had done any dissertation on the topic which is related to your topic, then please go through it, find research article related to it, read it carefully, read the conclusion, the limitation of the study and further studies which are required. By proper understanding of the limitation of the study, you can try to overcome the limitation in your study.
- You may talk with the experts in that field after taking permission of your guide.
- Before selecting any topic, please think about your career goals, if you want to go for further study and research after your masters, then you can select a topic in which you can do more work even after completion of your Postgraduation, you can do your PhD over it by doing research in deeper level but if you donot want to study after Postgraduation, then also you can choose an original topic.
- If you want to take your career graph higher, then please select such a topic which can be published in a good journal because it will help you a lot.

- Please select such a topic, which can be discussed and explained easily at any future interview. Select such a topic which can impress the interviewer.
- Please don't select such a topic, which is difficult to answer, or explain to your interviewer or examiner.
- Please think and identify your strengths and short-comings.
    - Think whether you are good in theory or practical work or patient interaction and dealing; and choose topic according to your strength.
    - If you are married, then think how much help you can get from your spouse and how much household work you have to do, select topic accordingly.
- Last of all, always be patient during selection of your dissertation topic, it is not possible for anyone to select a dissertation topic within seconds. So, if it takes time, please don't be frustrated, just calm down, search more articles, consult more journals, talk with your guide, seniors and select a topic which is good for you.

SOME SPECIAL CONSIDERATIONS

- If you are confused about choosing *in vivo* or *in vitro* studies, then one thing can be said without any hesitation that *in vivo* studies are always more relevant, because in *in vivo* studies, you are gaining important clinical data but there are multiple problems in *in vivo* studies-
    - To get sufficient number of patients with similar problem except dentinal caries, pulpitis, gingivitis or pericoronitis.
    - Similar treatment planning.
    - A wide number of clinical variables.
    - Willing patients for multiple recall visits in absence of symptoms.
    - Long clinical follow-up is practically impossible in 2 1/2 years.

   - Correlation between treatment and microscopic findings are really different.
- ❑ If it is an *in vivo* study, then think about the patient availability, whether it is possible for you to convince the patient for your study because patient consent is very important.
- ❑ Select such a topic where you can get the ethical clearance easily.
- ❑ In case of *in vivo* study, where patients follow-up is very important, then please think, how will you motivate the patient to come for checkup and recall visit even after complete cure or when they have no complaints.
- ❑ On the other hand *in vitro* studies have the following features:
   - Easier to start, do and end.
   - Factors are easily controllable.
   - Microscopic correlation is easier.
   - Clinical reproduction and result can be widely different.
   - Many limitations.
- ❑ Treatment comparison versus material comparison-
   - Treatment comparison encompasses wide number of variables even in *in vitro* studies.
   - Material comparison encompasses controlled variables.

- There are some studies which apparently look very simple and easy to do, but actual procedure is difficult and explainable result is difficult to obtain. For example:
   - It is very difficult to do a bond-strength study *in vitro* which will involve actual tooth-surface area. Normally, the Instron is considered the most common equipment to do a bond-strength study, but it requires far greater area to do a bond-strength study.

- *In vivo* bond-strength study can be done evaluating percentage of microleakage and long-term retention.
- Comparison between *in vivo* and *in vitro* studies is greatly hampered by presence of so many clinical variables i.e. salivation, temperature changes in oral cavity, masticatory forces etc.

- Microleakage: *In vivo* microleakage studies may be hampered by risk of permanent discoloration to the restoration and difficulty in measuring the gap in between material and tooth surface.
    - *In vitro* microleakage studies are dependent on the diameter of disclosing dye in the gap in between.
    - Efficacy in thermocycling in reproducing the temperature changes in the reproduction of leakage in the oral cavity is an area of concern.
- Questionnaire survey
    - The most important part is choosing the word of the question so that they can be understood by medical and non medical question alike.
    - If possible, the question should be in multiple choice quetions pattern, so that the time taken to fill the form will be minimum.

These are some examples of apparently easier but actually complicated studies, so before selecting a topic please consider all the factors which may cause difficulties in your work and then select the most suitable one.

Before the search ends, make sure you have the blessings of your parents and The Almighty in every step.

Be patient while searching do not get frustrated as tomorrow is another day, another beginning.

10

Monetary Grants

Funding Your Efforts

Vinayak Joshi

Outline of Topics Covered

- Introduction
- Acquiring of funds for research
- Unique research idea
- Matching idea with funding agency
- Writing a grant proposal

INTRODUCTION

One of the biggest challenges in doing research is getting the research idea funded. For any newbie with a research idea, getting some funds to carry it forward certainly acts as a motivation. For a decent concept to be developed, the associated researcher does needs some monetary support. This is where research grant is of great help. Having an idea need not always guarantee grants. There are certain set rules that one needs to understand and follow which makes that idea viable for some funding.

Currently, in India, there are numerous agencies that fund research ideas. It is one of the most common perceptions in India that research are not funded and thus are impossible to be carried out by individuals. Both the central government and the state governments have realized the importance of harnessing the indigenous talents. There are many grants available both nationally and locally which can fund an idea. Let us try to demystify the process of grant application. This chapter aims to explain you the simple way one can use to get the research idea funded.

ACQUIRING OF FUNDS FOR RESEARCH

Getting monetary funds for your research is just a simple three-step procedure that one needs to understand and follow:

Step 1: Have a unique research idea.

Step 2: Match your idea with the funding agency.

Step 3: Write the grant proposal.

Step 1: Unique Research Idea

One of the major criteria when seeking a monetary funding is that you have a good concept/hypothesis in place. Make sure that the research question in mind is well-formulated and is addressing an important issue. The funders are interested in funding a research idea rather than a research plan which is just a refurbished idea or a mere rehash of a known technique. If you think from the funder's point of view, you will understand that each funder is interested in solving a particular problem. As a grant seeker, you would need to identify problems within your community or patient population. The problems you are trying to find solutions should either solve some unmet need in that particular field or should be able to closely analyze the particular problem. One should only get into writing a grant when they have fully understood the problems, the limitations and have a proper plan of action.

There are many funding agencies and each of these funding agencies will be interested in funding only when you desire to solve a problem that matches with their area of interests.

Step 2: Matching Idea with Funding Agency

When your idea is ready to be put on paper in the form of a grant application, it is the right time to look for the correct funding agency which will suit your niche. Why would you need to do this matching? Well, each funding agency has their own research interests, thrust areas which they are interested in supporting.

When your research idea matches with their area of interest and when your vision promises some findings or results which they think that is worth investing, is when a grant is approved. It is not appropriate to write one generic grant application and use it for various different granting agencies. Each application has to be tailor-made according to the requisite of the funding agency.

After you have looked into the details, at the theme, interest and ideas of a particular granting agency and have understood the needs of the application, it is the time to get to step 3.

Step 3: Writing a Grant Proposal

Each grant application can vary, however there are certain parts which are common. Let us look into certain most essential and generic components of any grant application.

A grant application can be divided into following parts:

- ☐ Covering letter
- ☐ Table of contents
- ☐ Project summary or abstract
- ☐ Needs statement or need for the study
- ☐ Mission, goals and objectives or aims and objectives
- ☐ Project description
- ☐ Evaluation
- ☐ Biosketches
- ☐ Time lines
- ☐ Budget summary

- ☐ Budget justification
- ☐ Bibliography or references
- ☐ Appendix
- ☐ Other forms.

Each of the above could be included in a grant application. However, since the applications are tailor-made as per the requirements, one should only include what is expected or asked to by the granting agency. It is important for the applicant to remember that only the information asked should be provided. Any extra information which is not called for or with the intent of trying to impress on the funder could lead to the application being rejected. You should remember that the person reviewing your grant application may not have the time to go into all the extra details that you are providing, so make sure you stick only what is being asked for. All the parts of the grants are important in their own way, however certain points hold the key and those should be treated with extra care.

Covering Letter

Covering letter is one such point which needs some attention. This is the item that is first in the line of the grant application and will be read first by you grant application assessor. This is your chance to make a good first impression and convince the reader to look further into your application. Make your covering letter simple yet packed with enough power to get the evaluator interested in the application.

Keeping your covering letter brief you would want to start by introducing your institution. This will let the reader know where this is coming from. You should also mention about the community, population or the target group that is going to be part of this study. This should then be followed by mentioning something about the importance of the project you are about to undertake. At this point, make sure you are putting forth couple of the most important key points about your study that will highlight the study as well as generate the needed curiosity in the reader. You should also mention why you are applying for this particular grant with that particular agency or organization. This will tell the reader that you have fully understood the grant application which should be in commensurate with the objectives of the granting agency. Lastly, you should end the covering letter by thanking them for giving you the opportunity to submit the grant proposal. Make sure you have included all the needed personal contact information too.

Table of Contents

Table of contents (TOC) is also commonly known as content, guide to content or index, may seem to be simple and unimportant, but does play a vital role. The TOC should be prepared with specific attention not miss out on any item included in the grant. The TOC must include all the major headings in the same order as arranged in the proposal and include all that has been asked for by the funding organization. The TOC will act as a checklist for you to make sure you have included all the necessary information needed for the grant application. This will also help the grant reader to understand what you have included in the proposal. A busy grant reviewer may at times decide to check only the important sections of the proposal, and TOC will help in such situations. A well-formatted TOC, which ideally does not extend beyond one page, will help the proposal examiner to understand if you have paid attention to the minute details and have included all that is asked for, at a glance. In India, there are few occasions that the format of the grant application is not specific if a TOC should be included, in such case it is advised to add one, unless specifically mentioned.

Project Summary or Abstract

Project summary is also known as abstract, synopsis or project overview. Project summary no doubt is one of the most important parts of your grant proposal. It is the final summary of what your project is all about, concise in a page with a maximum of 500-600 words. This can tell your grant reviewer if you meet the necessary criteria for the grant funding. Considering your funder is a busy person, they may just look into the project summary and then decide if they have to look into the full application. If you have omitted any important information that they want or if your project lies outside the scope of the funders objectives, they may decide not even to review the full application. It is important to include all the core points in the summary. Hence, it is advised to write the project summary at the very end of your grant application, after you have structured the whole project. It would be a good idea to use the goals and objectives to build your abstract, which will make sure that the core points of your proposal, is included and abstract matches with what is written in the main grant.

Need for the Study

One of the important points that you always need to be aware of is that this section should be properly worded with attention on spelling and your sentence formation. Make sure that your writing is easily comprehended even by a person not belonging to your own speciality. Usage of simple language with commonly used words may be of help, especially when the reviewers are not from your own speciality. More than often the grant reviewer may not be from your own field. This section is where you get a chance to explain your hypothesis and try convincing the funder why you should be funded.

If your goals match with the goals of the funder to resolve a specific issue or trying to answer similar questions, then you stand a higher chance of being selected. This is where your proper matching of the grant application with an ideal funder comes to use. It is not enough to just have a big research idea, as ideas are not funded unless they are logical and rational. You will need to have clear vision and explain to them how you would try answering the research question, the short-term and the long-term outcomes that you foresee. For example, if the grant is from a local community, then your research should pertain to the issues you see at the local level. Only when the results of your study address either the problems or the welfare of the local community will your application have some consideration. Thc funder should see the potentiality to reproduce such results or bring it to some use in that local community.

For a national-level grant your question of interest should be addressing the concerns of the larger population, and how it will help answer the question or answer part of the larger question. Grant makers usually will consider when your problems address the needs of the community and when you are able to explain to them how well you will put the results to use. Ideally, the end result of any research should typically lead to solving other related questions or provide a solution to that question in totality. Funders are more interested when they see that your application is not just a one-time boom of a research interest and see the possibility of further continuation.

It is always helpful to back your plan and hypothesis using some of the data you have from another related study. It helps if you can make a comparison, for example the presence of HIV positive in your community as compared to that at a state or national level. Such comparisons help the grant evaluators to see the difference and can understand better the need for such a project in your community. Also the data from a pilot study is of great help to prove the grant evaluators that your claims about the probable result are soundly based on certain findings. It also assures the funding organization that you are serious about the project and that their investment will be in good hands. The funding agency always wants to play safe and grant the funds to well-established groups because of the proven track record of the funds being put to a proper and justified use. Always try to back up your claims with well-established data from other peer-reviewed literature, your own pilot studies and other relevant publications from your previous work.

Mission, Goals and Objectives or Aims and Objectives

Whatever it may be called, mission, goals, objectives or action plan, this is an important step in your grant proposal. This step elicits your understanding of the subject and how well you have planned this project. Here you will have to enumerate each major and minor step you would have planned for this project. You will have to detail out the major steps and the methods you would use to attain them. Every funder would be interested to fund only those ideas which are properly understood by the principal investigator and the funders should be convinced that the idea will be executed in necessary manner and is complying with their area of interest.

Writing a well-planned goals and objectives is your chance to convince the grant funder of your plans to apply the required methodology to obtain the correct results. An idea that is very well-planned, detailed and has achievable targets, has the highest chances of being funded.

Goals

When you write a goal, make sure that it is elaborate, explaining the funding agency what you exactly plan to accomplish. Goals would detail out the major steps you would follow to attain your target. Take the liberty to explain at this point what you plan to do, how you plan to do, what are the realistic timelines, who would do it and what would be the outcomes. Make sure that the goals you mention are realistic, concrete and are attainable. One should avoid making lofty and high-ended statements which seem unreal, for example "cure the world of pain" or "happiness to everyone in the world".

You are free to use flow charts or diagrams to illustrate to the funders your steps or ideas to carry out the project. All in all, this is your best chance to convince the reader of your ideas, so keep it clear, lucid and crisp. However, most of the grant applications in India do not have this section and only require aims and objectives mentioned, so just stick to what your application requires.

Objectives

After you have completed the goals, you will have to jot down the objectives. Objectives are nothing but the steps you would undertake to reach the goal. Completion of all of the objectives mentioned will help achieve the goal. Again, let the objectives be concrete and realistic. Objectives are the jigsaw pieces of the larger goal but each of these objectives should be treated as whole in themselves. Each objective should outline about what you are going to do, the methodology, how much or how many, or what is involved and the projected outcome. The Applicants are requested to follow the guidelines set in the application form. They should strictly follow and comply with the requisites of the funding agency and the above said instructions are just some generic guidelines.

Certain times the funders are not specific and at such time, the onus is on the grant writer to make his goals and objectives as clear as possible for the reviewer. Make sure you have just the right amount of objectives, too less or too many objectives would just indicate that you don't know what you onto or are just fishing for some results. Our experiences indicate that three objectives are what is very comfortable and can include all aspect of your research question.

Project Description

Every funder would like to know in detail about the project that they will fund. A funder will not just fund a good idea, if there is a lack of direction, if it does not progress growth, is not self-sustainable, or if it does not match with the funder's interest. The project description should clearly define the problem that is being addressed, the role played by you or your organization, the resources that you will contribute and the role played by the funder and how well it matches with their idea or theme.

The funder will only fund what they understand, so it is necessary to think from the funder's perspective. As a funder, they would be interested to know what is that they will accomplish by investing the money, what could be the return on investment (ROI) and what is that you can offer. A grant document is not just a scientific problem requesting money, but it should also be considered as a sales pitch, where you are trying to sell your idea. As a funder, they would want returns more than the "principal". They could measure ROI in terms of return per rupee or in terms of improvement for patients, organization, and community.

When you intend to write the project descriptions, make sure that it is clear, concise with as many non-technical terms as possible. Usually, the person reviewing your grant may not be from the same background so if your grant is very technical then try avoid difficult words such that a lay person will be able to comprehend your description. It is always a good idea to let some of your friends or colleagues who are not in the same field as you, read your research project to find out if they can comprehend it.

The project description will usually includes all the major events and should be in a logical order as described in the goals and objectives. Although your project description is built around the goals, you should remember to be clear and concise.

A project description includes material and methods, the resources available to conduct the study, the timelines and the description of the execution of the project, the roles played by various persons involved. It should also include the contribution from your organization in terms of infrastructure and resources, the plans for evaluation and one of the most important of all, dissemination of the data or information.

Certain funding agencies will want to fund only if the institution has the needed expertise and the resources available to them. They would also try to make sure that the institution is also chipping in its share in form of equipment, personnel, can independently carry out a certain parts of the project and are not entirely depending on the grant funds.

Make sure you have covered all the major points about the project. At times, it may be necessary to understand or research about the funding agency to exactly understand what they need so that our project matches up well with it. Try using simple, commonly used words, try explaining in layman terms any technical process or words and follow a uniform pattern for naming, designating or numbering to avoid confusion to the reviewer.

Always have your goals and objectives ready before you attempt to write the project description. Try to follow the guidelines set by the funding agency. You may also want to read it a couple of times to examine the project from various angles and try explaining in advance anything that may look unusual in your projects. This helps your project document to be properly structured and well-packed. Try looking into it from the reviewers point of view, which might also help you secure some of the loose ends. This is your best chance to tell the funders why your project should be funded, so tread carefully!

Project Evaluation Report

When funder and you look at the same problem, is when the research grant gets funded. Once a grant is funded, the funding agency has made its investment into your idea for the possible solution to that problem. Every funder who has invested, would be interested to know the progress and the cumulative end result. They would want to make sure that the project is headed in the same direction and the same pace as promised. As a grant seeker, it is necessary for you to have an evaluation plan in place.

At times certain grant necessitates that you report to them on a regular basis of the progress of your project. This is where your setting of timelines during the formulation of goals comes into play. For proper reporting, it is important that you document every step that is detrimental to the results of your project. Proper documentation will help you in preparing an effective evaluation report.

During the course of your project, if you encounter any situations wherein you would want to change your original plan, then it is necessary that you inform the funders and only make the changes with their consent. As they have invested the money in your project they have the legal rights to know of any changes that would be made to the project. They are your partners in this project. The evaluation report serves two purposes: (i) to understand the progress of the project and to make any necessary changes in it if necessary as you progress (ii) to understand the outcome, if it was a success or effective to which extent.

Biosketches

The funders who would fund your grant idea would want to make sure that the funds are in capable hands. There could be a very well written research project but if the team is not well composed then the project, may not succeed.

When writing the biosketches, please remember that this is not the usual resume that one would use for jobs. This should be a one-page document which will mention what will be the role of each person in the project. It should clearly mention who are the key persons in the project. The biography will include the name, the rank, the job title, speciality of the person, experience that is relevant to that research project, degrees, professional activities like membership with different societies, job descriptions and a summary which will detail relevant experience or similar projects in the past. Make sure you have an able team, which will justify being in the team. A team with relevant past experience and accomplishment will certainly give the funders the confidence and may be one of the important elements in your proposal getting funded.

Timelines

This is a graphical representation of the important time points in the study. This can be presented in a graphical format using a table or a graph. Often times this is also called as Ghat chart. The timeline should note all the major milestones in the project. You can use the goals and objectives to make note of the important milestones in the project. Make sure you list all that you plan to accomplish at each time point, however make this entire look very realistic and keep away from making unattainable claims. If the project is for 3 years, the funder may want to know how you have planned this project and what you would be trying to accomplish every six months or in a year's time. The funder may also want you to send six monthly or annual reports so setting realistic time points is very important.

Budget Summary

Most of the grant application needs you to give a budget summary. In this, you are not just stating the overall cost of the project, but also giving an itemwise budget. It is pretty important that you clearly state what will be the contributions by your organization and by any partners that you have. Contributions to your organization and by your partners can be both in kind or cash. This will also help to re-assure to the funders that only they are not liable in this project and that you have an equal share. No funder would be happy to know that you will entirely depend on their funding to carry out this project.

Utilization of the facilities at your center (electricity, water, computer, software, books, etc.), the manpower in the form of employees, office and laboratory supplies, utilization of existing equipment, all such can be included as the contribution from the grantee or partner organizations. The funder would be interested to know what will be your liability for this project and how much you are committed to this project. It also may help to assure the funders that you would be able to sustain without their help in the future. This promises the funders of the long-term benefits of funding such a project.

Based on your goals and objects, you can list all the items that are going to be part of the project. Take into the account all the direct costs, indirect costs, miscellaneous costs in form of office supplies, the cost of traveling, wages, transportation and so forth. Missing out any of the items means that your organization would be liable to bear the cost, it is advised that you take the time to make a detailed list.

When you are setting the budget, make sure you are realistic. Never try to understate the cost trying to impress on the funder, nor try overstating your budget. The funder must have done his homework and you would not want to be caught on the wrong foot at this stage. It is advisable to get the real costs of each of the items as existing in the market at the given time; this will help to keep the budget real. Certain grants also want you to divide the budget for each year (for multiple year projects). Each year budget may also be divided into a certain percentage of the annual budget for non-consumables and consumable goods. In all these situations, your budget planning should tally with your major time points and goals which were mentioned earlier.

Budget Justification

The funder who is funding your project will definitely be interested in why and how you would be utilizing the funds. All the items should be listed and a justification given as to why they are needed in that particular project. One should understand that different grants have different budget allocations. In some of the grants there may not be any funds for travel or books, some grants have no budget allocation for equipment, some grants are only for the development of infrastructure, and some grant has just money for consumables. So depending on the budget limits and the restrictions applied by the funder in terms of certain percentage or budget limit you should make your item list and give valid budget justification. If the grant is a multi-year project like a three- or four-year project, the funder may ask for a year by year budget distribution.

Each year budget may then have certain budget allocations for consumables, equipment, or infrastructure or travel depending on the granting agency. Your budget planning should not only follow the major milestones and the goals but should also accommodate the budget allocated each year by the funders. The justifications for the expenses should be realistic yet accommodate all the needs. Sincerity would surely payback here.

Along with sincerity, one should also be logical. Normally a three year research project would have need of grant funds more in the first year, which will lessen the second year and with least the third year. The reviewers of the grant will certainly look into this. However, if a grant has equal funds allocated each year, then the above example doesn't hold true. Budget justification also allows you to explain certain points which you were not able to accommodate during the project summary or need for study. However, avoid being repetitive. Once you have listed all the items and have explained their need in the study, you are almost done. It's time to move one of the last few steps to wrap-up the grant application.

Bibliography/References

All the research papers or books or any online document you might have referred in preparing the proposal, should be cited in this section. Citations give an authentic feel to your proposal, shows how well you have read, if you have included the recent materials, which is a sign of how well-researched and new your idea is. Citing the documents also protects you from plagiarism. Do avoid cut-paste jobs when preparing your application. The reviewers may consider this very seriously and will definitely not be in your favor. It is advised to read the scientific materials and then utilize the data given in there with your own sentences then resorting to shortcuts.

Another point that you can think of is to include as many of your own or from your team-mates research articles as citations. This will prove to the funders about the experience and authority that you or your team has in this particular area. This will help when there are other competitors applying for the grant are from the same specialization. You can also use the materials given on the funder's website; use any research articles or publications from the funders to make the funders understand that your application is a close match to their central theme or area of interest. For example, if you are writing a grant for a department of science and technology, then your application should speak about how it would add to the existing science or technology, or utilize the existing technology to answer existing lacunae.

Also, one should take care to adhere to the citation style as required by the application form. If not mentioned, one can go with Vancouver system as it's one of the most commonly used citation style. Using a reference manager would also help and save time setting up the bibliography. Some of the commonly used reference managers are Endnote, RefMan, Mendeley, and Zotero. These are available both as paid license version and free open software.

Appendices

For every grant this section is very important. This section helps to keep the body of the grant application limited to discussing only the core issues. If you are limited in space for project summary, need of study, project description or time lines, then you can add additional documents as appendix. Make sure you have mentioned the relevant appendix numbers in the body of the application. Appendices can also be used to provide detailed information regarding your organization, the infrastructure available, organization or study flow charts and the equipment and their technical specifications and other information available. This section can also be used to provide the detailed bio sketches of the key personnel and detailed list of relevant publications, organization registration or recognition certificates, letters from partners or work done at your organization.

However, unnecessary information should be avoided as the reviewers do not have all the time and always remember to make it easy for them. Please stick only to the that information that the grant application has specified. Trying to impress the funders by providing more information than necessary may also act against you. Appendices should be properly numbered as indicated in the application and arranged accordingly so that locating them should be easy.

Other Forms

Lastly, you will have to fill the forms which are provided with the application. These forms may be different with each of the funding agencies. The forms can be anything from a questionnaire you would have to fill about your organization, or maybe a brief summary of your intended project. Certain state and national agency require you to get these forms notary attested or take an undertaking of some kind. You should remember that you are to follow the funder's requirements at all times during your application procedure. All applications should be custom-made according to the need of a funding agency and in doing so all other things discussed above become secondary.

Ready Reckoner:

When you have any research ideas begin with matching your ideas with a suitable funding agency.

↓

First Step in your application procedure
Start with: Need for Study.
Make sure your research idea matches with the main theme of the funding agency

↓

Write the Mission Goals and Objectives; this is vital for your further steps. This should be based on your need for study; accomplishing the idea which you had.

Contd.

Next step would be Project Description. This step needs that goals and objectives to be completed. The materials and methods should elaborate on how each major goals/objectives are achieved.

Timelines comes next and this based on the objectives and the project description. Here you need to specify the time needed to meet each major goal/objective. Take into to consideration time needed for each based on the material methods and protocols. The time line should take into consideration the time required to achieve each of the goals enumerated earlier.

Next follows Budget summary and Budget Justification. Both these are based on the goals, objectives and timelines given above. Be realistic.

At this time go with selection of who would be in your team. Make the necessary Bio-sketches as recommended above. Biosketches will justify each person's role in the project.

Have a colleague or a friend from other field read the document. Make sure a lay person can comprehend your project. Pay attention to grammar and spellings. Have uniform font type and size. Most commonly used are Times Roman and Arial. Use page numbers.

Have all the Appendixes ready for all the above. Number them and arrange exactly as used in the main application.

Time to get the Bibliography or References in place. Make sure you follow the exact styling as required. Follow a uniform pattern. Double check the reference details like volume, page number, year, to avoid mistakes.

This is the time to write the Project Summary. Please note if any word limit is in place. Follow the guidelines.

Contd.

↓

Table of contents; Make sure you double check the page numbers listed here.

↓

Finish your grant application with the much needed Covering Letter.

↓

Have a colleague proof read your entire application. Pay attention to all the signatures and attestation needed. Enclose all the required documents. Enclose required number of copies of the grant. Some grants need that you send a soft copy version in a CD/DVD. Have your application completed and checked well before the deadline.

↓

Send the application and keep your fingers crossed!

11

Delivering an Effective *Viva Voce*

Seema Anjenaya

Outline of Topics Covered

- Introduction
- Merits of *viva voce*
- Demerits of *viva voce*
- Approaches to viva
- Group viva
- Sample set of viva questions

INTRODUCTION

Viva voce is a Latin phrase literally meaning "with living voice" but most often translated as "by word of mouth". It is a face-to-face interview of the candidate, by the examiner during evaluation process. The oral assessment or *viva voce* is a component of many undergraduate and postgraduate examinations in medicine. It is commonly used technique for testing student's knowledge, confidence, reasoning and analyzing abilities. It thus forms an important tool of assessment.

The oral examination has often been criticized for being very subjective and being influenced by the learning and bias of the examiner. Framing questions is an art and requires wisdom on the part of examiner to extract the correct answers from the students. Vivas are traditionally conducted by preferably two examiners—an External and an internal examiner. They should normally consult before the examination about who is going to ask about what, however this does not often happen and there are rarely clear guidelines about what it is fair to assess and what not. The major issues related to conduct of viva voce are validity, reliability and fairness.

Thus, strategies need to be developed to improve the oral examination or *viva voce,* as it has its own merits as a tool of assessment. Apart from testing in-depth knowledge, it can be also used to assess confidence, communication skills, decision making, problem solving etc., which may not be assessed by other modes of assessment.

Let us see the merits and demerits of *viva voce* and what strategies should be adopted to make it a valid and significant assessment tool.

MERITS OF VIVA VOCE

- Apart from testing higher levels of cognition, it can also test attitude, skills, professional competence and communication skills.
- Provides valuable and immediate feedback to the student, teacher and the teaching learning process.
- Provides flexibility of examination to deviate from standard pattern when required.
- Provides opportunity to the student to defend his/her statements, enables the students to express their ideas and voice their opinion on the subject that is asked.
- Allows quick evaluation covering a wide area of the syllabus.

DEMERITS OF VIVA VOCE

- Undue anxiety and mental fatigue in students may interfere with a student's performance and will not give a true indication of his or her ability. Their understanding or capacity to think critically can be limited due to anxiety.
- Bias: Examiners may be influenced by students' accent, dress, gender, social background, etc.
- Students from vernacular medium who have difficulty in speaking English are often judged on language and vocabulary rather than knowledge. Also, a student who speaks fluently may score more, though his content knowledge may be poor.
- Lack of anonymity: Examiners inevitably know whom they are examining.
- Can get affected by subjectivity and personal bias of the examiners
- May lack validity, reliability if questions are unsuitable and ambiguous and the marking system is arbitrary
- Retrieval of the evaluation is difficult
- Can be time-consuming, especially if large numbers of students are examined.
- There could be variability in the time spent by examiners in assessing each student.
- Students with hearing or speech difficulties may require some adjustment to the assessment process.

APPROACHES TO VIVA

Traditional

It is usually found to be unplanned and influenced by subjective factors.

Objective Structured Approach

It is a systematic, planned, organized and controlled approach, with minimum subjectivity and maximum efficiency and effectiveness. If the examiner follows these steps, it would result in better examination which would test predetermined objective catering to all levels of learners.

Steps for Objective Structured Approach to Viva

- Develop viva question bank covering full syllabus topics and subtopics.
- Validate questions in advance by an expert team.
- Structure the topics into subtopics to carry out detailed examination on vital points covering "must know", "desirable to know" and "nice to know areas".
- Quality of questions: They should be clear, grammatically correct, unambiguous, with a mix of open-ended, closed and leading questions.
- Preferably make four to five questions in proper sequence on a single topic, starting with easy question and subsequently to higher level of questions which test understanding.
- Ensure that there is no repetition and overlap of questions.
- Prepare standard marking pattern; separate marking may be done for the content matter and for other factors like confidence, communication skills etc.
- Appoint sufficient number of examiners, so that at least minimum two examiners can examine the candidate at a time to eliminate bias and subjectivity.
- Call for an advance meeting of the examiners and brief them about the quality of questions, standard-marking pattern etc.
- Coordinate viva with written examination.
- The *viva voce* should last for 10–15 minutes.

For Examiners

- To relieve student's anxiety.
- To treat the students as adult learners. Do not insult the students by passing offending and personal remarks.
- To ask questions preferably from the viva question bank provided.
- To proceed from easy to difficult and from general to specific questions.
- To ask appropriate questions in proper sequence and deviate when required.
- To stick to the time and marking pattern.
- Marking should be done by each examiner independently and an average of marks may be taken at the end.
- Isolate already examined students from the students yet to be examined.
- Offer short breaks during lengthy oral assesments.

Other Strategies

- Making and storing audio or video recordings of *viva voce* if feasible, which would enable retrieval of the evaluation whenever necessary.
- All areas of competence specified for the exam, (e.g. diagnosis, problem solving, management, communication skills, ethics, etc.) must be explored.
- Faculty development: Teachers should be trained for conducting a structured, valid and reliable viva.

GROUP VIVA

Another method of conducting viva voce is by "group viva", wherein it may be conducted in a group of 5–10 students at the same time **(Fig 11.1)**.

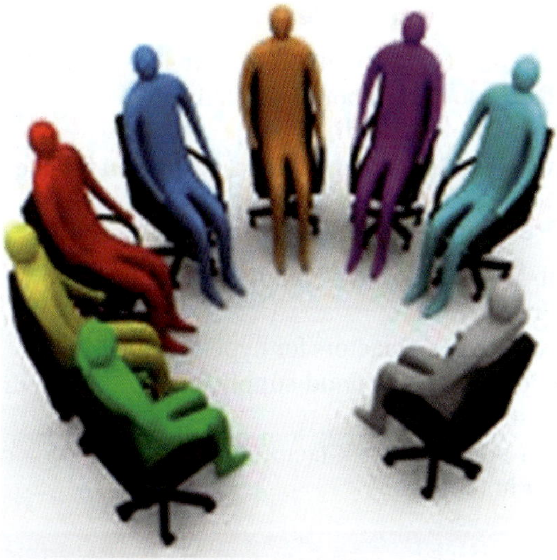

Fig 11.1: Group viva

Advantages of Group Viva

- It helps to relieve student anxiety.
- It allows the students to appear for viva as well as to listen to questions asked to other students and to learn from their mistakes.
- The students get training for viva, which helps to improve their performance during subsequent individual viva.
- Large amount of content can be covered in a short time.

SAMPLE SET OF VIVA QUESTIONS

The questions asked by the examiner to students during *viva voce* should be clear, precise, short, unambiguous, valid and preferably covering all topics.

Defective Framing of Question

- Tell us something about BCG vaccine?
- What do you know about hypertension?
- Describe the stomach?
- What do you think about cervical cancer in females?

Right Framing of Question

- What is the dose and mode of administration of BCG vaccine?
- What are the risk factors for hypertension?
- Give the relations, blood supply and lymphatic drainage of the stomach.
- Tell us about the risk factors and screening for cervical cancer in females?

CONCLUSION

Viva voce is an important tool of evaluation and should enable to give feedback about our teaching and also about the student's level of performance. Instead of discontinuing the use of oral assessments, ways should be identified to improve the reliability and validity of the oral assessment.

The examiner-student encounter should not be confrontational, but rather comfortable. It should aim to find out what the candidate knows rather than what he does not know. The viva voce should end positively. It is also important to prepare the panel for the viva, with mandatory pre-viva meetings to discuss requirements and expectations, as well as approaches to questioning. The validity and reliability of oral examinations can be increased by the use of structured approach, by training examiners, increasing the examination time, number of examiners, number of topics examined and taking an averaged item scores.

Objective structured approach towards viva makes it

efficient and effective tool of evaluation. There is a need to develop viva voce management system which requires conscious effort on the part of teachers and curriculum planners.

REFERENCES

Shukla Das, V.G. Ramachandran, Sonal Sharma. Oral Assessment (Viva voce'), chapter 26. In: Pritha S. Bhuiyan, Nirmala N. Rege, Avinash Supe. The Art of Teaching Medical Students, 3rd ed. Elsevier.2015; 321-329.

Anshu. The Oral Examination, chapter 15. In William P Burdick. Principles of Assessment in Medical Education, Jaypee. 2012; 166-172.

Tejinder singh. Oral Examination (Viva Voce), chapter 19. In: Tejinder Singh, Piyush Gupta, Daljit Singh. Principles of Medical Education, Fourth ed. Jaypee. 2013; 117- 122.

12

Technology and the Postgraduate Student

Keeping Abreast with Times

Ajay Kakar

Outline of Topics Covered

- Pacing up with new trends in technology
- Searching textual data
- MEDLINE
- Systematic reviews
- Photographic documentation
- Data processing

PACING UP WITH NEW TRENDS IN TECHNOLOGY

Technological progress has been advancing at a rapid pace. Over the past century, the pace of this progress has increased exponentially. Technological change today is so rapid that a complete makeover of how information is handled takes place in lesser and lesser time. Concepts, machines and equipment today have a much smaller life span than in the past. A very poignant example is the laptop, computer and the mobile phone.

New models barely get established and a paradigm shift in technology renders them obsolete in less than a decade. Analog cameras which ruled the roost for over six decades are now completely extinct. They have been completely replaced with the digital camera and now a huge component of the digital camera is almost extinct due the incorporation of the digital camera into even the most entry-level mobile phone. One excellent source for how technology is progressing is the book "Megatrends" which kind of predicts the trends which are moving human lives in various directions.

Education has also been impacted in a similar fashion by technology. The core requirement for education is "information" and a place where collated information is easily available. The term "library" has been very strongly impacted with "information technology". A young teen today probably has not found the need to visit a traditional library for getting any information as part of his/her education. Education, specifically in the healthcare area, depends extensively on the latest information on any scientific advancement that has taken place. Healthcare education also very strongly needs documentation in the form of text as well as in the form of images.

Retrieval of existing information from around the world has now completely gone digital and so has documentation and record keeping. Not only is the case description and finding become digital so has the photographic records. Publications which form the essential source of all information have also gone digital. Even though the large majority of publications in the form of journals and text books are still published on paper, all of them will also have a digital version. A few have already made the shift into only digital versions of the publications.

Postgraduate (PG) education, especially in the health-care sector is extremely dependent on information. The requirements for information can be broadly categorized into the following:

- Needs for basic knowledge on the subject in general.
- Needs for information from the examination point of view.

- Access to information for the purposes of compiling a dissertation as a part of the program.
- Article publication as part of the PG program.

The internet has today become the defacto standard for all of the above. As mentioned earlier, all of this information is processed digitally now. The digital information can be again split into three different formats. These are:

- Textual information.
- Digital photographic information.
- Numeric data which can be subjected to statistical analysis.

SEARCHING TEXTUAL DATA

All of the above is very strongly dependent on the "internet". Any and every student is today completely aware about "Google". In fact, it is has become synonymous with a search engine. Factually, there are many many more search engines available on the internet, but "Google" has become so popular due to its intensive marketing that the term "googling" has come to mean carrying out a search on the internet. Even though the Google search engine is a great tool and provides fantastic information on almost any kind of topic or subject, the data generated can be from any source. This information is not necessarily always authentic. A search engine will throw up any links and browser pages, which have the keywords being searched.

The information may have been posted by nonprofessionals; could be personal websites; could be an amateur hobbyist putting up information; or can be general information on the subject posted by association for educating the lay person. Search engines will not usually filter information specifically required for a scientific inquiry. Pages generated by a search engine have to be shifted through and takes up a considerable amount of time and effort. Other than Google, other search engines to be considered are yahoo.com, bing.com, altavista.

com, ask.com, AOL.com etc. Even though, most of the data generated from different search engines is more or less the same, at times other engines may come up with some useful additional data. In any case, Google dominates the search engine market with more than 80% of all searches being done the world over.

All of the above search engine pages will only provide a basic and very wide set of data, especially for a PG student who is searching for very specific, narrow and relevant information. Most scientific information is mostly available in journals and publications from societies and associations. This is supplemented by periodicals, newsletters and textbooks which are not always available online in its full form. There is a universal method of indexing scholarly articles and this process is automatically done when the article is published in a peer reviewed indexed journal. The most accurate and very specific information is obtained by looking into these indexes. This index is maintained by the United States National Library of Medicine (NLM) and is titled as MEDLINE.

MEDLINE

The MEDLINE (Medical Literature Analysis and Retrieval System Online, or MEDLARS Online) database comprises of life sciences and biomedical information including bibliographic information for articles from academic journals covering medicine, nursing, pharmacy, dentistry, veterinary medicine, and healthcare. It contains more than 21.6 million records from over the 5,500 publications covering biomedicine and health from the year 1950 onwards. Earlier the MEDLINE database covered articles starting from the year 1965, but this was enhanced and retrospective citations as far back as year 1950 were added to the main index. New citations are continually added to this database on a daily basis.

Originally the MEDLINE database could only be accessed by special terminals installed in libraries and the printed results of the searches were handed to users by the librarians. All of this completely changed when the internet explosion hit the world around the year 1996. The graphic browser on any Windows based computer or the Macintosh suddenly allowed users to access all kinds of data. The NLM created a special portal to let browsers directly search the MEDLINE database. The best past is that this search was completely free. This portal is known as PubMed and the URL link to be used on any browser is *www.pubmed.com* or *www.pubmed.org*.

This portal searches the entire MEDLINE database and generates the list of citations and abstract of all the citations. Occasionally a full article is available for downloading if the publication had given such access rights for the downloading the entire article. In any case all full articles are always available on payments. MEDLINE is today the best possible resource for any health-care scientific online search to be carried out. Full articles are also available to members. Membership IDs and passwords or access rights are often available for PG students through universities who have agreements with NLM.

Other than the MEDLINE which only accepts data from indexed journals, there is one other useful search method which generates relevant and specific information for scientific research purposes. It is called Google Scholar and is a free to use search engine accessible with the URL link "*scholar.google.ca*". Google Scholar focuses on scientific and hard-research academic material that has been scrutinized by scientists and scholars. The content includes graduate theses, legal and court opinions, academic publications, medical-research reports, physics research papers, economics etc. This is definitely a very useful tool for reviewing the literature for any proposed study or research topic.

SYSTEMATIC REVIEWS

One new area of data assimilation that has become possible recently due to the open search engines has been the aspect of systematic review of the literature. A systematic review of the literature is an excellent methodology for PG students in the health sciences to be able to do a library theses or even a complete paper or as part of the regular dissertation in the PG program. MEDLINE is the best resource for this kind of work. Postgraduate students should log into the pubmed site and generate a list of all citations with the appropriate keywords. The keywords are completely dependent on the subject matter being researched. The optimal choice of keywords is the first step in this process. Once the list of citations has been generated, an abstract for each of the citations can be viewed and there is no cost attached to his process.

The abstract will definitely carry the title of the publication, the journal, date and author details and will usually have a synopsis of the aims and objectives and a short conclusion on the results of the study. The data on MEDLINE is so vast and extensive that even the most obscure of topics generate 300–400 citations. Reading and collating so many full articles is impractical and arduous. The abstracts allow easier reading and will filter down the appropriate articles to numbers that are easily manageable. Once the abstracts are short listed and access password can be obtained from the university to get the full articles and make a complete review of literature.

PHOTOGRAPHIC DOCUMENTATION

One very critical element in PG studies, especially in the health sciences is documentation of cases, specifically photographic documentation. Photography has undergone a complete revolution, specifically in past two decades. The first change was the move from analog to digital media, which means that the photograph, instead of being recorded on a negative and then being transferred to a colored positive was now recorded as a digital file on the camera on an electronic media. This digital file could be replicated and copied an infinite number of times on any other digital media like the hard disk of a computer. Simultaneously, there was the advent of various media types to store digital data. The very popular floppy disks of the 1990s had given way to the compact disc (CD) Drive and then the digital video disc (DVD). But these media were also short lived. They soon were replaced by a very easy to carry and rewritable n number of times USB drive. The earlier drives had a limited capacity to store data, but even the limited capacity was much more than that of a floppy drive and almost the same as a CD and soon enough equal to that of a DVD. Rapid technological enhancement has today given us USB drives of very large capacities. These allow almost a complete library to be carried around on a small (1 cm by 2 cm) electronic chip housed in a plastic body.

With this huge amount of real estate in terms of storage space available very easily, the file sizes of various forms of data also grew in size. Since this discussion is on digital photographs the discussion will be restricted to image files. Fortunately or unfortunately, there are just too many formats in which a picture file can be stored. Also the picture file can be stored in any resolution. Even though true from a certain view point, that the higher the resolution the clearer the digital image, this has a certain limit since the human eye can only discern objects to a certain point. If the resolution gets higher, the image becomes difficult to visualize. Digital cameras have made it possible to store very high resolution images, but these high resolution images become cumbersome and bulky to process especially when a big number of pictures have to be worked upon. For example. even copying about 50 very large resolution images from one drive to another could easily take more than 7-8 minutes. Opening an image of this kind could easily take a slightly slower processor-based laptop more than 2-3 minutes. These are extremely long times for image processing.

Image files can be digitally stored in over ten dimensions. These dimensions are usually measured in width by length in terms of pixels. A very basic image is generally 640 pixels wide by 480 pixels length. This size is fine for a video display but not the greatest for making a printed postcard size photograph. Other image resolutions are 800×600 pixels, 1024×768 pixels, 1280×960 pixels, 1536×1180 pixels, 1600×1200 pixels, 2048×1536 pixels and so on and so forth. Of these, the size of 1280×960 pixels is more than adequate for any requirements of case documentation or publication. It is easy enough to digitally process and make great picture of even 8 inches by 10 inches.

One last aspect is the format in which digital images should be stored. There are a number of image format files possible. A few of these are "jpg", "png", "bmp","tif", "raw". The digital world can get quite formidable and unwieldy at times. It would be beyond the scope to discuss these file format. It would suffice to say that the most widely used and easy to manage format is the "jpg" file type. This is the file type that should be used by PG students for digital image processing.

DATA PROCESSING

Software technology has now also eased the process of data management and analysis for all kinds of health science studies. The most strongly recommended tool for this purpose is the "Excel" spreadsheet. For PG students who are electronically inclined, a short course on Excel will pay rich dividends. Data can be easily entered into an Excel sheet. Once populated, the spreadsheet offers a wide variety of statistical computations in an instant. Not only are the statistics available, the data can also be used to present graphic charts in multiple formats for easy viewing and processing. It is highy recommended that PG students get familiar with the spreadsheet as part of their PG education.

This concludes the various aspects in which technology has touched the health sciences and made it possible for study of the health sciences much more easier, wider and more definitive.

Index

Page numbers followed by *f* refer to figure.

D

E

N

P

R

S

T

U

V